HULTON PRACTICAL TEACHING SERIES

Primary Gymnastics

Brian P. Callington

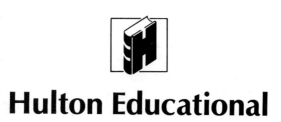

Hulton Educational

First published in Great Britain 1985
by Hulton Educational Publications Ltd
Raans Road, Amersham, Bucks HP6 6JJ

Text © *Brian P. Callington* 1985
Illustrations © *Hulton Educational* 1985

ISBN 0 7175 1310 6

Artwork and cover design by Anna Hancock
Edited and designed by Charlotte Rolfe
Photographs by David Bell

Phototypeset 11/12 Linotron Times
by Input Typesetting Ltd, London SW19 8DR

Printed in Great Britain by R. J. Acford, Chichester.

Contents

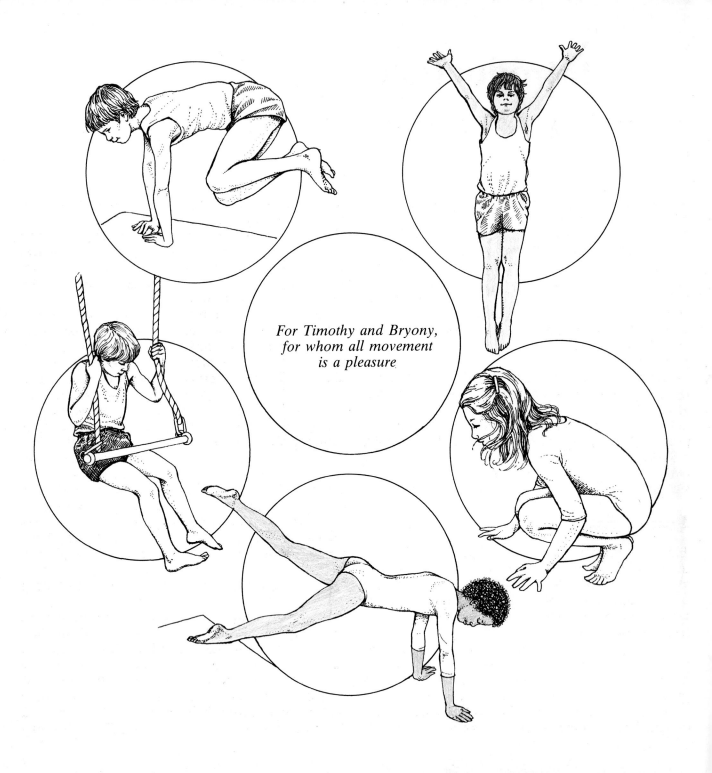

*For Timothy and Bryony,
for whom all movement
is a pleasure*

Introduction

All children in the primary school love their gymnastics and games lessons but for many teachers these sessions, particularly in gymnastics, can be an ordeal; the nature of the work, the environment and the apparatus involved present their own unique problems. This book seeks to relieve teachers of these worries by providing guidance in the organization of lessons, ideas for the development of the work and, most important of all, abundant material for immediate use in a programme of educational gymnastics.

The book is directed in the first instance towards teachers of the primary age range, but the activities and suggestions for organizing material and developing ideas could be included in work for older pupils. Wherever it is used, it is hoped that the book will enable both children and their teachers to enjoy and profit more fully from their involvement in this subject.

About the book

This book is both a source of activities and ideas for teachers to use in educational gymnastics lessons and also, for those who wish to use it as such, a comprehensive and developmental programme of work suitable for classes throughout the five to thirteen age range.

The first part of the book contains brief sections offering advice and guidance in those areas which need to be considered by anyone developing a programme of work in this subject. This is followed by the activities section. The activities have been designed and arranged on a thematic basis as this is the traditional approach to teaching lessons in educational gymnastics.

Twelve broad movement themes are identified which cover the full range of movement experience. In each of these themes, activities and ideas for work are given for use in each part of a lesson, namely, the introduction or warm-up, the floorwork, the apparatus session and the conclusion. Selections can be made from these activities to build up single lessons or a whole series of lessons within each theme. To explore movement ideas fully and to allow children to progress towards skilful and confident gymnastic performance, several lessons need to be devoted to each of these twelve themes.

Success in gymnastics, as in most subjects, is achieved through continued practice and the slow development of ideas or concepts in the work. Children must therefore be given ample time to practise and to achieve success in each activity, with new ones only being introduced to develop movement ideas or to create completely different challenges through a change of direction in the theme. If the activities contained in this book are used in this way the resulting programme will certainly extend to a full year of work, whatever the age of the children being taught.

All of the activities in the book are given titles in order to distinguish them and to highlight their different concern with movement forms within a theme. Many of the introductory and concluding activities within each theme take the form of gymnastic games. Children particularly enjoy starting and ending their lessons with a game and these activities have this appeal whilst still retaining their link with the movement concerns of the main theme activities. However, activities within the floorwork and apparatus work sections of each theme, which will form the main body of work in lessons, are designed specifically for the development of skilful gymnastic movement, and this must be the focus of concern at all times for the teacher during these sections of a lesson.

Concepts and skills in educational gymnastics

In this book, gymnastic movement has been categorized into themes under headings such as 'Movement on the feet', 'Curling and stretching', 'Shape in flight' or 'Movement in flight', work tasks have been presented within these themes in forms which require the children to think for themselves, for example, 'Move with only one foot touching the floor' or, 'Find three high stretched shapes'. In this way, attention is focused upon the nature of bodily movement and children are able to discover for themselves the many ways in which different movement forms can be represented. This approach to the teaching of gymnastic skills allows all children to achieve a degree of success in all aspects of the work. Some children may show more imagination, others may be more spectacular, but all are able to develop movements to satisfy the broad requirements of a particular task – something which is highly desirable in what for many pupils is quite a difficult subject.

Reference to formal gymnastic skills is unnecessary and should be avoided within the main theme work of educational gymnastics lessons. Movements which approach such formal skills as a handspring, a headspring or a walkover might well emerge in the children's work and if so they should be developed through attention to such elements as speed, shape and general control. However, there is no need to give such movements specific names, for once this is done they assume a quite new importance. Formal gymnastic skills are very refined and

stylized movements, and they are seen by the children as such. Many children can become discouraged through the introduction of formal skills work as they begin to view their own movements as poor handsprings or poor walkovers rather than as the original movements which they probably are. If formal skills are to be taught within a theme of work then they should be left until the last lesson in that theme and be brought in as a concluding activity. To use them earlier is to risk discouraging many pupils by placing them in a situation of failure and this can significantly influence their overall confidence in the work.

To encourage children to discover gymnastic movements for themselves through the exploration of concepts and ideas within a particular movement theme and to then develop these by considering factors such as body shape, speed and balance in the work benefits not just bodily control, it also challenges the children's mental capacities. Gymnastic skills and routines which are developed in this way are not only enjoyable for the child to perform, they are also very pleasing for the teacher as they contain that very special quality of originality which is so nice to see in all children's work.

Lesson planning

The activities in each of the movement themes in the book are grouped in the same way under the headings, *Introductory activities, Main theme: floorwork, Main theme: apparatus work* and *Concluding activities*. This follows the accepted format for lessons in gymnastics and the activities which are used in each of the four parts of a lesson should satisfy quite specific objectives, as follows:

Introductory activities These should occupy about one sixth of the total lesson time and should act as a preparatory warm-up for the children. This is essential in establishing the right physical and mental condition in pupils for the work to be done in physical education lessons. The introductory activity does not have to relate to the main theme of the lesson, although it is beneficial if it does.

Main theme: floorwork The main theme of a lesson should always be introduced through floorwork activities as the children can experiment freely with movement ideas at a basic level, without the complications and worries which can be a feature of apparatus work. For example, in 'Movement on the feet' children can be asked to find as many ways as possible of moving on their feet and a wealth of ideas will emerge whilst the children are working on the floor. However, many of these movement forms will quickly disappear when the children transfer onto the apparatus where feelings of insecurity will suddenly predominate. It is essential therefore that children experiment fully with a movement idea through activities on the floor in order to establish an understanding of how the idea can be interpreted and also to build up control and confidence in their performance. Subsequent work on the apparatus will reflect the amount of thought and practice given to floorwork activities. These activities should account for about one third of the total lesson time.

Main theme: apparatus work Again this section accounts for about one third of the total lesson time. It allows for the ideas and movements conceived in the floorwork activities to be developed in a completely different and more challenging context. For example, rolling movements which the children may find relatively easy on the floor suddenly become very demanding when they have to be performed along, across or around apparatus. The understanding of ideas and concepts introduced in the floorwork can be reinforced through further emphasis in the apparatus work. This is particularly well achieved with concepts such as balance and smoothness in movement which can be critical to the successful performance of apparatus routines. In the case of certain themes, movement ideas can only be properly tested or fully realized through the introduction of apparatus. This applies particularly to themes concerned with flight, where the extra height to be gained from jumping off apparatus provides the time so vital to the performance of movement in the air.

Concluding activities These should be used during the final one sixth of lesson time. The end of a lesson is the time for the children to unwind from the mental demands of the main sections of work. This can be achieved by using a fun activity based upon the work of the main theme or by completely changing the nature of the work with the introduction of movement ideas to be met in the next theme to be covered.

It is the practice in many primary schools for the younger classes to have their gymnastics lessons on the same morning or afternoon in order that the apparatus can be left out. Where this occurs introductory and floorwork activities should not be neglected; the children can still perform them in the floor space around the apparatus, or space can be quickly created by moving some of the free-standing pieces of apparatus to the side of the room. On occasions when more floor space is required for these parts of the lesson, as is the case for work in the 'Flight' and 'Take-off and landing' themes, a degree of pre-planning will be necessary to arrange for the floor space to be clear of apparatus. Some form of common syllabus or work schedule for infant classes is recommended, since this ensures that apparatus arrangements satisfy the needs of all.

Lesson management

The guided discovery approach to learning, which is fundamental to educational gymnastics, allows for quite a free working environment. However, for children to benefit fully from this approach, certain considerations need to be made with regard to the management of lessons. A basic feature of the educational gymnastics lesson is that all the children should be able to work at the same time, but for this to happen successfully the children need to be constantly encouraged to work independently and,

3

in particular, to avoid queuing, something which happens all too frequently around apparatus. The development of children's spatial awareness is vitally important to this form of gymnastics teaching. It should be encouraged and receive constant attention from the very first lesson.

If pupils are to develop a wide repertoire of gymnastic skills it is important that they be given ample opportunity to explore movement ideas within each theme covered and the time to consolidate, through practice, the skills learnt in a lesson or particular activity. Activities can be changed far too quickly, before the majority of a class have gained anything worthwhile from the work. This can be guarded against by using the children's achievements in the work, rather than any time factor, as the criterion for deciding when to change.

Because of the rather abstract nature of many of the concepts and terms used in gymnastics work, for example 'points of balance' or, 'the smooth transfer of body weight', specific directions need to be given not just before but also during the actual performance of an activity. It may even be necessary to keep up a running commentary to highlight the points which the children should be considering and to draw attention to the different interpretations of a movement idea as they appear in the pupils' work. Such comments, coupled with a constant observation of the children working, are essential, both for safety reasons and to determine whether activities are being performed satisfactorily. Children who satisfy activity tasks particularly well should be asked to demonstrate their work to the rest of the class, as this will stimulate thought in the others.

Quality of work produced by the children should always be the uppermost concern in a lesson and the teacher's knowledge of the pupils in a class will determine what are acceptable standards of performance. It is particularly important in educational gymnastics to urge pupils to be self-critical and to strive to produce work which they themselves consider to be good, as there are no standard skills by which performances can be measured.

The time for moving on from one movement theme to the next depends largely upon the children's standard of work and their general understanding of the various concepts that have been presented. However, it is important to guard against boredom; the interest of the pupils in the work is critical in motivating their learning and this must be given due regard when considering whether to continue with a particular theme or to introduce another. Pupil enjoyment is a key objective in every lesson; if the children enjoy the work then they will be motivated to try new ideas and to work for optimum standards.

Use of apparatus

Apparatus work forms an integral part of every gymnastics lesson and is crucial to the development of the ideas and movement principles being promoted within the main theme. As with all apparatus in a school, gymnastics apparatus serves as a teaching aid, providing a further medium through which the children can manipulate and develop skills. For some, it will facilitate the breakthrough in their understanding of a particular movement concept. This is to be seen with the concept of balance where many children move onto apparatus and adopt hanging positions which they mistakenly believe to be forms of balance. For most children, however, the apparatus offers an exciting means of developing ideas formulated in the floorwork activities, giving the opportunity to try out movements in a new and challenging situation.

Apparatus arrangements should first and foremost satisfy the needs of the work theme being covered, serving to develop the movement concepts contained within that theme. To be effective the apparatus must offer a variety of challenges, even where it is of the same essential nature. For example, in the rolling and balance work, which requires flat-topped apparatus, surfaces of different lengths, widths and even gradients should be provided.

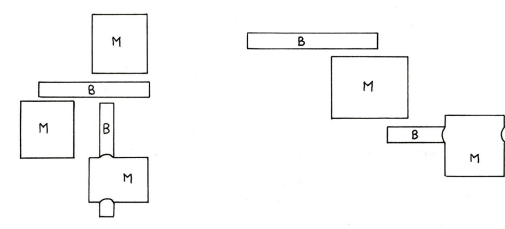

Use benches (B) in twos or even threes in an offset pattern. Arrange mats (M) to allow for work in a variety of directions. Where appropriate, drape mats over benches to encourage a wider range of movement.

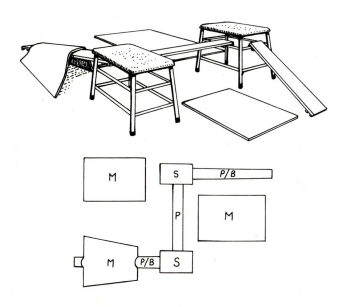

Benches and planks (P/B) in conjunction with stools (S) provide inclined and higher work surfaces.

In deciding upon the apparatus to be used particular care must be taken to ensure that it will encourage the children to experiment with movement ideas, rather than to just 'play safe' in their work for fear of falling and hurting themselves. Where necessary, surfaces should be well padded both for working and for landing on, and at all times the height of apparatus used must be appropriate to the age and the ability of the children.

If there is insufficient apparatus for everyone to have room to work at the same time, activities should be modified to include use of the surrounding floor space. For example, activities which require two movements on the apparatus can be changed to include one movement on the apparatus and one movement on the floor, so allowing two pupils to use the apparatus alternately.

It is very important to realize that apparatus arrangements can often condition the thinking and the movement of children, rather than promote original ideas and activity. A good example of this is in the queuing which happens at apparatus. Whilst the teacher is discouraging the pupils from doing this, the position of the mats around the apparatus could be encouraging them to queue by suggesting a correct route for moving over the arrangement. Mats should always be positioned with this point in mind and in a way that will encourage movement onto and off the apparatus in a variety of directions.

When movement ideas are transferred from the floor to apparatus it is advisable to ask the pupils to work, initially, on a single piece. This allows them to gain confidence in working on the apparatus and to concentrate fully upon developing the ideas without being overwhelmed by the many movement possibilities offered by a large arrangement. Having successfully transferred their work to a single piece of apparatus, the children can then be encouraged to try their movements on other pieces, both to explore the movement ideas even further and to experience the different demands made upon them by the various pieces of apparatus.

The final watchword on apparatus use, and perhaps the most significant in terms of safety, is that *chasing games should never be played using large apparatus.*

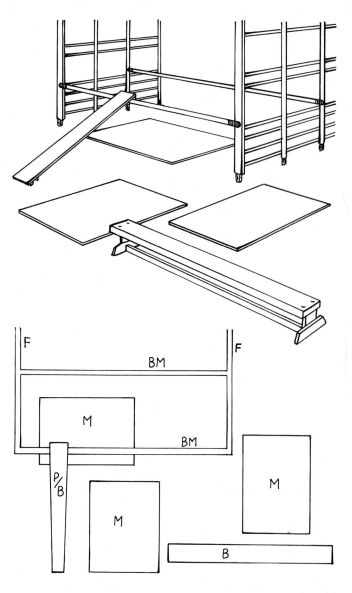

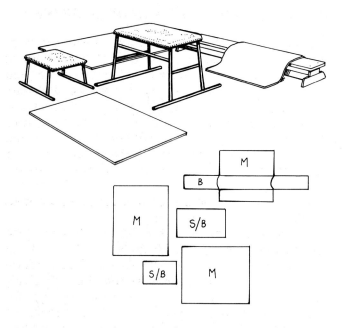

Stacking stools and boxes (S/B) used together provide similar work surfaces, but of differing heights and sizes. Padded benches can be used to extend such arrangements.

Beams (BM) and climbing frames (F) can be used in conjunction with other apparatus to encourage movement in and out of the enclosed spaces they create. Additional apparatus extends movement possibilities and allows for a larger number of pupils to work around these fixed pieces.

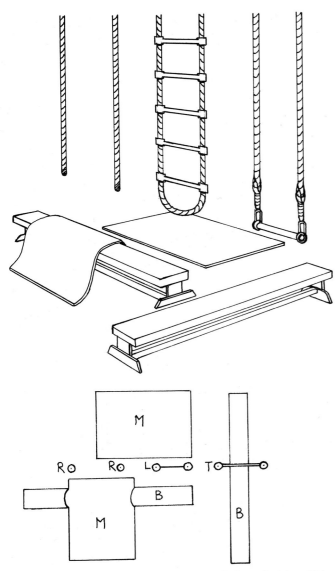

Hanging apparatus such as ropes (R), a ladder (L) or trapeze (T) can be linked with free-standing apparatus. This will give younger children greater mobility to develop a range of movements. The dangerous practice of swinging on hanging apparatus will also be discouraged where pupils are required to include movements on adjacent, free-standing apparatus.

Sequence work

The essence of gymnastic activity is the ability to perform and link together individual movements and skills in the form of a sequence. For this reason sequence activities appear towards the end of the floorwork and apparatus work sections in all the movement themes in the book. Sequence work provides the opportunity to combine ideas and skills from different parts of the programme and to draw on and reinforce the various principles which have been covered in each of the themes in a more meaningful way. Children will better understand why it is important to have control in landing, to maintain body shape through a roll or to hold a balance nice and still when these are elements in an ongoing movement routine.

Partner work and group work

Whatever the age of the children, these forms of work require a reasonable degree of proficiency in any given movement theme before they can be used to worthwhile effect. However, children do enjoy working together and simple partner activities can be introduced at quite an early age. These can take the form of simple matching exercises where the children copy one another in performing shapes or very basic movement routines. Partner support movements and sequences where one child bears the weight of another should not be used, however, until much later in the junior years.

Group work activities should also be reserved for the top junior age range. The qualities of spatial and body awareness need to be well developed before three or more children can work together effectively on a group movement task where the object is for pupils to combine or synchronize their movements in a floorwork or apparatus routine. The children also need to be proficient in the particular movement skills to be used in the routine and to have had a lot of experience in working one with another on different partner activities.

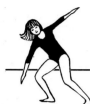 # Movement on the feet

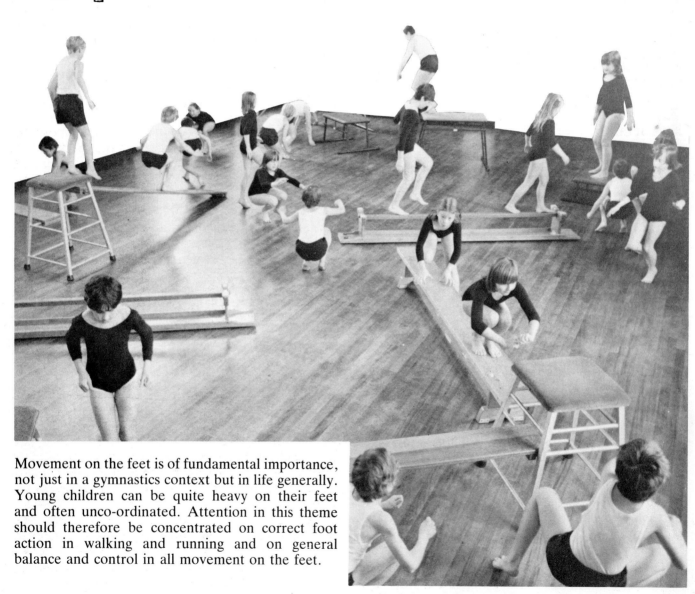

Movement on the feet is of fundamental importance, not just in a gymnastics context but in life generally. Young children can be quite heavy on their feet and often unco-ordinated. Attention in this theme should therefore be concentrated on correct foot action in walking and running and on general balance and control in all movement on the feet.

Introductory activities

These activities should require the children to change pace and direction in their movement.

1. 'Stuck in mud'

Choose one or two children who must chase and try to 'tag' the other members of the class. Pupils who are 'tagged' have to stand still with their legs apart until they are 'released' by another pupil crawling between their legs.

2. Circular run

Ask the class to sit in pairs, each pair in a space and to number themselves one and two. All the number ones should then sit with their legs tucked in tightly and on a signal from the teacher all the number twos get up, run once around every pupil who is sitting down and then return to their partner. When all have finished, the number twos can then sit cross-legged whilst the number ones do the running. To encourage the children to move quickly, ask to see the first pupil to get back to his partner.

3. Lose your partner

Working in pairs, one pupil stands at arms length behind his partner and on a signal from the teacher the child at the front tries to shake off his partner by running and dodging whilst the one behind attempts to stay that close. When the teacher calls 'Stop', the children must stop immediately and they can them check which of them has been the most successful in their particular task. Partners can change places for each run.

4. Moving to space

In this activity the children have to move about the floor trying to stay as far away from each other as they possibly can. When the teacher calls 'Stop', each pupil should be in a space sufficiently large that they cannot touch anyone else. The activity should first be performed at walking pace but as the children get better at finding and moving into space the speed of movement can be increased to a run. With each stop, the children's attention should be drawn to the empty spaces around the floor and the areas which are too crowded as this will benefit their general spatial awareness in the activity.

5. Circling a partner

Working in pairs, one pupil sits in a tucked position whilst the partner, on a signal from the teacher, has to run around him three times in one direction and then three times in the other direction. To encourage the children to move quickly the activity can be treated as a race by asking to see the first pupil to finish seated, with their hand raised. The partners should take it in turns to sit and to run.

More changes of direction can be introduced into the activity by instructing the children to change direction whenever they hear the teacher clap, and to finish only when they have managed to complete three successive circuits in one direction.

6. North, South, East, West

For this activity the children all sit in spaces and face the same way. Using the signals North, South, East and West to indicate the four walls of the room, the children then have to walk in the direction called by the teacher. As an alternative to this the children can be asked to face the North wall continually and to walk backwards and sideways when moving in the other three directions.

The activity can be made even more demanding if a large hall is being used or, if the pupils show good directional sense and spatial awareness, by asking the children to jog. In this case, it is important that changes of direction be called out quickly.

Main theme: floorwork

The first activity used in the floorwork section of all lessons in this theme should stress the nature of foot action in carrying body weight, such is its importance to posture and general mobility. The first three activities offered in this section are all included because they lay particular emphasis on this point.

1. Walking slowly

In this simple activity the children merely have to walk as slowly as possible in any direction and stop on command. Whilst they are moving about attention should be drawn to the heel to toe action of the foot in walking and the children can be asked to feel how their weight passes through the foot, starting at the heel and passing down the outside edge of the sole.

2. Walking a narrow bridge

Imagining that they are on a very narrow bridge, the children must walk normally but as carefully as possible and in a straight line. Emphasis should be on how the feet must stay in line and be placed very carefully with the heel leading the movement. Balance, using the arms, is also important to this form of movement, and attention can be drawn to the part that the arms play and how the head must also be kept still.

3. Tightrope walking

Ask the children to walk an imaginary tightrope.

In this form of movement the toes play a far more important role as they make first contact with the floor. The children should be encouraged to feel for the rope with their toes before putting their foot down.

In both this and the previous activity use should be made of any lines marked on the floor, or the

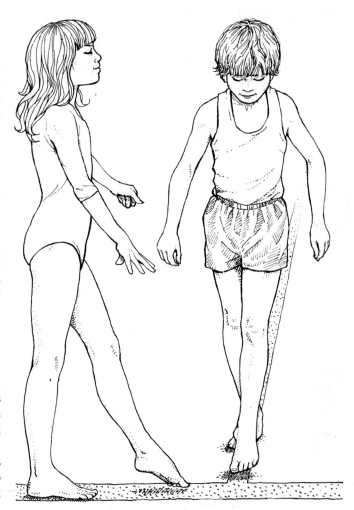

Tightrope walking.

strips of wood which make up a block floor, to assist the children's accuracy in foot placement. The children might also be asked to perform the activities with their eyes closed as this would focus their attention even more upon the feel of the movement and the way the foot must take the body weight whilst also maintaining balance. This would be most safely achieved with the pupils working in lines and moving across the floor together.

10

4. Running

This activity embodies several factors concerned with movement control on the feet, and a different one can be emphasized each time the children run. The basic activity is that the children run about in any direction, avoiding each other and trying to stop as quickly as possible when the signal is given.

(i) Quietness: Ask the pupils to be as quiet as possible in their running. The point to stress to the children is that whilst they cannot change their weight, they can seem lighter and be much quieter when they run if they cushion their footfall by bending the leg and 'rolling' their weight through the foot from the heel to the toe, rather than landing flat footed.

(ii) Running on the toes. Ask the pupils to run on their toes and to consider if this is easier than normal running, if it is more tiring, if it seems natural and if it is easier or more difficult to stop.

(iii) Balance: Running requires considerable balance, particularly when changes of direction occur. For this activity the children can be asked to run about as before but also to change direction each time the teacher claps, in this way changes can be effected very rapidly. Ask the children to feel what they do to change direction in their running, to feel what part the feet, arms and the rest of the body play.

(iv) Control in stopping: Stopping quickly involves extending the leading leg and sinking at the knee to absorb forward movement. This is best illustrated to the class by asking someone who has shown that they can stop instantly to do a demonstration. The other pupils can then try this at half pace running.

The practice of stopping when moving at speed can be developed to include changes in direction. The technique of using the 'braking' leg as a spring to thrust the body into a new direction enables quite substantial changes to be made, with turns through ninety degrees being possible. The pupils can try this whilst moving at jogging pace with changes again being directed by the teacher clapping a signal.

5. Movement in different directions

To develop general foot control and awareness of foot action in moving, ask the children to walk sideways and then backwards and on each occasion to consider the following questions: Which part of the foot touches the ground first? Is it easier or more difficult to stop than when walking forwards? How do you stop? Do you lose balance more often than when moving forwards? Are there any other problems?

6. Movement in different ways

Ask the children to find different ways of using their feet to move about the floor.

The movement forms most likely to appear are hopping, skipping, crouched walking, bunny hopping and jumping. Jumping is an activity which merits separate attention in another theme but consideration should be given to the other movement forms which emerge. Hopping and skipping in particular merit attention as these are skills which require co-ordination, balance and a high degree of general control.

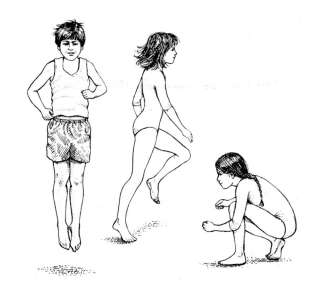

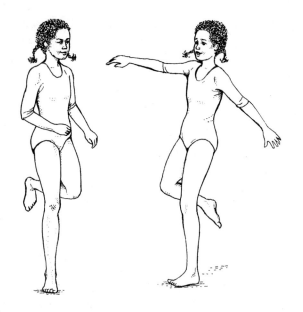

7. Hopping

This skill can be explored and developed through a series of exercises.
(**i**) Ask the children to hop first on one foot and then on the other. Is it easier on one foot than the other? Are there any other differences?
(**ii**) Ask the children if they can hop backwards. Is this easy?
(**iii**) Can they hop sideways? What are the problems here?
(**iv**) Place hoops around the floor and ask the children to hop in and out of them, using each foot and trying not to touch the hoops. Ask the children what problems they find with this activity and how they keep their balance in the movement.

8. Skipping

The approach to this skill can be the same as that used for hopping. Can the children skip backwards and sideways? Ask them which parts of the foot they use. Can they skip slowly? Can they turn and can they stop easily when skipping?

Main theme: apparatus work

SUITABLE APPARATUS: Benches. Upturned benches. Benches inclined at a low level. Low platforms and boxes.

Initially only low apparatus should be used in order to minimise the children's worries of falling and to allow them to remain safely upright when working, without the need to use their hands. The apparatus should also, ideally, offer different lengths and widths of surface on which to work as well as gradients to move up and down.

1. Move along please

In this activity the children move freely about the different pieces of apparatus and at each piece they step on and walk forwards along it. The children should be encouraged not to queue or to stop at all but to keep moving to where there is space on or around another piece of apparatus.

This activity can be repeated with the children moving sideways and then backwards along the apparatus.

The previously emphasized points of feeling for a surface with the feet prior to taking body weight, quietness in moving, the need for balance and the part played by the rest of the body in maintaining general control can all be featured in this activity.

2. Move in different ways

Ask the children to find different ways of moving along the apparatus using only their feet.

The forms of movement used in the floorwork activities are likely to reappear here which will allow for the points made then concerning balance and control to be re-emphasized. These will have particular significance if the movements of hopping and skipping are attempted on the apparatus.

3. Movement combinations

This activity serves as an introduction to the development of movement sequences around a piece of apparatus.

Ask the pupils to move around the apparatus and to walk along each piece of apparatus that they come to but to travel between them using different forms of movement on the feet. If the class perform this activity well, showing good control in their movement, the alternative can be tried of walking across the floor and using a different form of foot movement to travel along each piece of apparatus.

4. Sequence around a piece of apparatus

For this activity each pupil works on a single piece of apparatus to develop a movement sequence in which they travel along the apparatus and across the floor, each time using a different method of travelling on the feet.

Initially this sequence can be of just two parts, along the apparatus and return across the floor, but it can then be extended and developed as follows:
(i) To include three and then four parts, the latter involving two movements each on the floor and the apparatus.

(ii) The pupils could be asked to include particular movement forms in the sequence, for example a backwards movement or a hopping movement. The task might eventually be to use specified forms of movement for each part of the sequence.
(iii) Ultimately the children should be left to develop their own sequences as a test of their imagination and movement skill. At this point the teacher should merely put an upper limit on the number of parts to the sequence and advise upon the suitability of movements where pupils appear to be having problems.

5. Sequence around the apparatus

The sequence work of the last activity can be developed by allowing the pupils to work around two or three pieces of apparatus and eventually by letting them move freely about the room. However, the sequence should be limited to a given number of parts, probably six at the most to include three movements on the apparatus and three on the floor, otherwise the children will have difficulty in remembering and repeating their movements and this will influence the overall standard of the work.

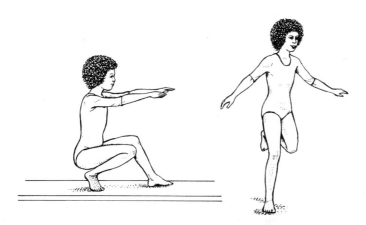
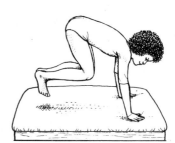

Possible sequence using two pieces of apparatus.

13

Concluding activities

1. No touching

In this activity the children move around the floor and try to avoid touching each other. The speed at which the children move can be directed by the teacher. This will affect their rate of success. At first the children should try the activity at just a slow walking pace and this can slowly be increased to a run.

As the final activity in a lesson this can be used as an elimination game with those pupils who touch having to sit out or line up ready to change.

2. Distance hopping

In this activity the children count the number of hops it takes them to cross the floor. If they lose control and stumble or touch the floor with the other foot they must start again. Designate a start line and a finishing line for this activity. Do not have the children hopping up to a wall as this can be quite dangerous if children should stumble or fall into the wall.

3. Hop, step and jump

From a standing start on one leg the children can try to complete the sequence used in the triple jump athletics event, seeing how far they travel across the floor. The children should all work in the same direction across the floor.

4. Sharks in the sea

This is a useful game for getting the mats put away.

The children walk or run between the mats and on the signal, 'Sharks in the sea' they have to move onto a mat. Allow only two pupils on a mat and remove one mat after each call until only one remains. Pupils failing to get onto a mat are eliminated.

5. Statues

The teacher stands on one side of the room and the pupils on the other. Whilst the teacher's back is turned the children walk across the floor, but when the teacher turns around they must stand perfectly still and any child seen to move has to return to the far wall. The child who manages to cross the floor first is the winner.

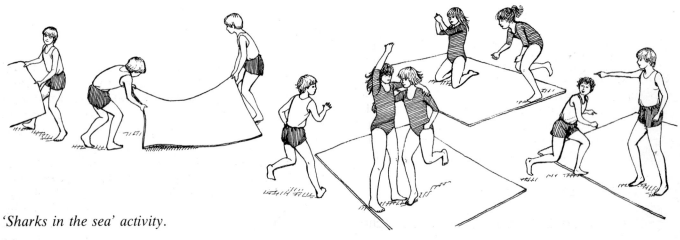

'Sharks in the sea' activity.

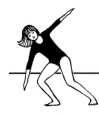

Curling and stretching

In gymnastics work children tend to forget about the limbs that they cannot see, so attention should be paid in this theme to the individual body parts and to achieving the fullest range of movement in all joints. In all stretching work the children should be asked to think of their feet and hands as points.

Introductory activities

1. Run and stretch, run and curl

In this activity the children run about the floor and on the signals from the teacher 'Stretch' and 'Curl' they stop their running and assume an appropriate shape.

2. Stretched and tucked

The children first walk about the floor on their toes with their bodies as extended as possible. They then move about in as tight a tucked shape as possible. Having practised these two shapes and ways of moving, the children can then move about the floor as they wish, but on the signals 'Stretch' and 'Tuck', the movement must continue with the body stretched or curled up, as indicated by the call.

3. Bridges and burrows

For this activity half the class adopt stretched shapes in the form of high bridges and the other half crouch into tucked positions. Both groups then move about the floor with the 'tucked' group passing under the 'bridges'. The children should try to avoid touching each other and on the signal 'Change', the two groups exchange positions.

4. In and out

In this activity the children work in pairs with one child adopting a high 'bridge' shape and the other, on a signal from the teacher, passing under this bridge, around a pillar, back under the bridge and around the other pillar in a figure of eight pattern. Whilst performing this movement the pupil must also try to avoid touching the bridge.

This activity can be performed a given number of times by each partner and to make the movement a little more vigorous the teacher could ask to see the first person to finish seated, with their hand raised.

5. Over and under

In pairs, one child crouches in a tucked position and the other stands with legs apart. On a signal from the teacher the standing child walks over his partner and then crouches, whilst the partner now stands and walks over the top. The children should not touch each other as they pass.

This activity can be used in a limited space but with the floor free can be performed with the pairs progressing across the floor from one side to the other and then back again with the children walking backwards.

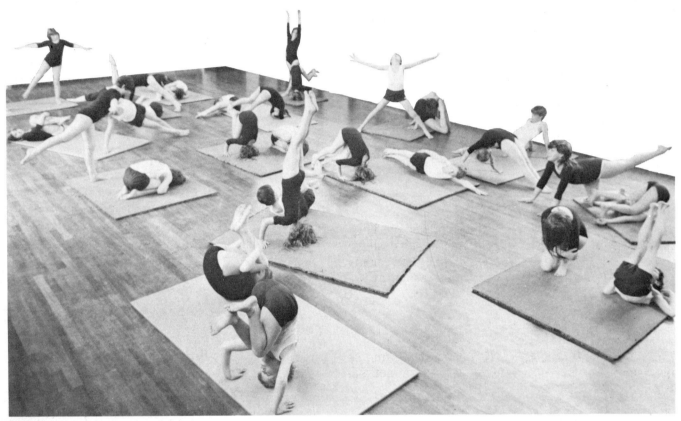

Main theme: floorwork

1. Different curls

To explore the many curled shapes that are possible the children can try different ways of curling up their bodies to make tight shapes. If the children work in pairs they can pass a hoop over each other to check if all the limbs are tucked in and to find which is the smallest shape.

2. Curl and stretch

Ask the children to move across the floor or a mat by using alternate stretching and curling movements.

An idea could be given such as moving like a caterpillar, but the children will find several ways of satisfying the task, and giving suggestions does tend to condition the thinking of some pupils.

3. Stretches

Ask the children to find a position where their bodies are stretched as much as possible. After holding this position for a while, they should find a different stretched shape. Attention can be drawn to each limb in turn whilst the children are holding a shape to check that it is fully extended, that all joints are

16

stretched and that they have 'points' instead of feet and hands.

Through this activity the children can be asked to perform:

(i) Wide stretch shapes.

(ii) Long, thin stretch shapes.

(iii) High and low stretches.

(iv) Arched or 'bridge' stretch shapes.

The same attention to detail can be given in each activity and the pupils' attention can be drawn to the interesting variations to be gained by working at high and low levels.

4. High and low

Ask the children to perform a stretched shape lying on the floor and then to perform the same shape standing. The children can then see how many shapes they can find that can be performed at the two levels.

5. Symmetry

The older pupils who are familar with this term can be asked to find symmetrical and asymmetrical stretched shapes.

6. Stretch and curl floor sequences

Ask the children to perform a stretched shape and to then move through a curled shape into a different stretched position.

Attention to detail should be the same as in the previous activities with the added concerns for control in the movement and 'flow'; the pupils should try to make the transfer through the movements as smooth as possible.

This sequence activity can be considerably developed by increasing the number of shapes to be included and by asking the children to work out different sequences based upon combinations of high, low, wide, thin, arched, symmetrical and asymmetrical shapes.

Main theme: apparatus work

SUITABLE APPARATUS: All the usual gymnastics apparatus is suitable for work within this theme.

In all the apparatus activities attention to detail in the shapes performed should be the same as in the floorwork activities, with the children being reminded to curl tightly or to fully stretch their limbs.

In each of the first five activities in this section, where the children are exploring ideas for curling and stretching on the apparatus, it is advisable to let them work out their ideas on several different pieces as they will then be better prepared for the later activities which allow for general movement around the apparatus.

1. Curl on

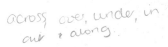 across over, under, in out & along.

Ask the children to find as many curled positions as they can which they are able to perform on top of the apparatus.

2. Curl around

Ask the children to find different ways of curling around a piece of apparatus.

3. Curl under

Position mats under the apparatus and ask the children if they can get into curled up positions hanging under their apparatus.

4. Stretch covers

Ask the children to find as many stretched shapes as they can which cover as much of their apparatus as possible.

5. Different stretches

In this activity the children explore the different ways of using their apparatus to adopt stretched shapes and try to find as many different stretches as possible.

6. Stretch and curl apparatus sequence

Ask the children to develop a sequence of two stretches and two curls using both the apparatus and the floor space around it.

Attention in this activity should be on control and smoothness of movement as well as aspects relating to shape. The children should also be made aware of safety factors in transferring from the apparatus to the floor: they should move smoothly, and if jumping off, should do so only onto their feet.

As in the floorwork, sequence work on the apparatus can be considerably extended by asking for particular forms of stretched and curled shapes in the movement. All the different forms of stretched and curled positions referred to in the earlier activities could be requested in this sequence, together with items relating to symmetry and work level.

7. Around the apparatus

Ask the children to move from piece to piece of apparatus by travelling in a stretched or a tucked shape across the floor, or by using combinations of the two, and at each piece of apparatus to perform both a stretched shape and a tucked shape which can be either on or around the apparatus.

After performing this activity satisfactorily the children can be allowed to develop their own stretch and curl sequences to include different pieces of apparatus. A limit should be imposed on the length of these sequences as children will quite happily continue to add movements and then find it impossible to repeat their routine. A limit of six movements to include three pieces of apparatus is appropriate for older juniors only.

Concluding activities

1. Caterpillar race

In this activity the children move across the floor 'caterpillar' fashion by stretching forward and then pulling themselves up onto their hands and knees. Using this technique the children can move quite quickly and can race across the floor.

Variations on this form of movement which the children might also try include:
(i) In a press-up position with hands and feet only on the ground the children have to move forward by walking their feet up to their hands and then their hands out away from their feet.
(ii) Lying on their backs with their feet together the children use their feet to push themselves across the floor.

2. Duck walking

The children squat on their haunches and whilst maintaining this position they have to walk across the floor by bringing their legs around the sides of their body.

Either working in teams or individually the children can race across the floor using this method of travel, but care must be taken as the exercise is very tiring.

3. Circle a partner

This is an activity which should be reserved for the older junior pupils.

Working in pairs, ideally with a larger pupil and a smaller pupil working together, the smaller pupil starts on his partner's back and tries to move from there, right around the front and onto his partner's back again without falling off. The supporting partner must try and help him to get around as best he can.

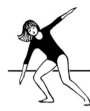

Twisting and turning

Younger pupils need not be worried about the difference between these two forms of movement, but older pupils should understand the difference as they are capable of more precise movement and should discriminate between the two in developing their movement sequences.

Turning is the total movement of the body around a particular axis. In twisting, part of the body turns whilst the rest remains still, turns the other way or follows the initial body turn rather like a corkscrew.

The body can be turned in a variety of ways about three axes:

1. Longitudinal axis, enabling movements such as spinning on the feet or knees and sideways rolling in a stretched position.
2. Transverse axis, giving movements such as forward and backward rolls.
3. Medial axis, which is through the middle of the body from the front to the back and which facilitates turns such as in a cartwheel.

Turning is quite a difficult movement concept for children to understand, and it is very helpful to briefly discuss with them what things they can think of which turn. If, as is likely, the children describe such things as wheels and the hands of a clock then these can be used for encouraging different ideas and movements in the various activities.

Emphasis in this theme should be on control, both in the performance of twisting and turning movements and particularly in landing or stopping after such movements.

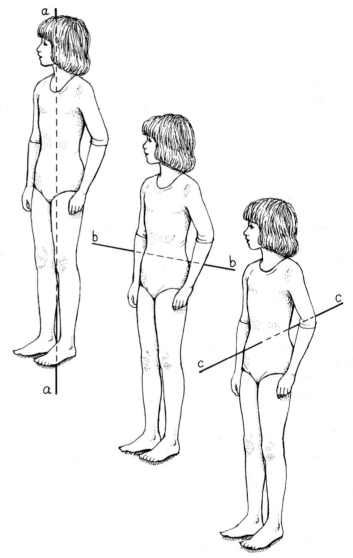

The three axes: (a) longitudinal, (b) transverse and (c) medial.

Introductory activities

The activities in this section are all particularly useful for encouraging the development of spatial awareness in younger pupils.

1. On parade – walking

Start this activity with the children standing in spaces near to the centre of the floor. From this point the children then walk in the same direction towards one side of the floor. The teacher then gives the commands 'Turn to the left', 'Turn to the right' or 'Turn about', and the children must walk in straight lines and try to obey by turning as directed.

2. On parade – standing

In a limited area the previous activity can be used, with the children standing in a space and merely turning on the spot according to the teacher's commands.

3. Walk the straight line

In this activity no commands are given by the teacher but the children may only walk in straight lines up or down the floor. They must stop, to avoid bumping into each other, but may only turn left or right through ninety degrees when changing direction. If there are lots of lines marked on the floor, the children could be asked to try following these.

This activity could be used several times with the children walking at faster speeds.

4. Stop, look, turn

The children run freely about the floor until they are told to stop, which they must try to do instantly. The teacher then gives the instruction to look left and right to decide which of the two directions is the best change of course to take, the pupils then turn the appropriate way and move off again when told to run. The children do not have to run in straight lines but they must turn through ninety degrees when choosing a new course.

When the children become proficient in determining quickly the best change of direction to take the calls can be reduced to merely 'Stop' and 'Run', and ultimately these calls can be replaced with just a clap to signal a change of direction.

5. Stand up, sit down, turn around

This is another activity which can be used in a limited space and which requires the children to move quickly and correctly according to the teacher's directions. These directions can be of the teacher's own choosing and could include commands such as 'Turn around', 'Sit down', 'Stand up', 'Onto your backs' and 'Onto your fronts'.

Main theme: floorwork

1. How can we turn?

From a standing position the children try different ways of initiating body turns. The following methods may appear but can otherwise be encouraged:
(i) Use of the feet in merely walking round.
(ii) Jump turns, the turn being initiated in the jumping action.
(iii) Throwing the arms or a leg in order to generate a spin turn.
(iv) Turning on the feet by pushing the body around with the hands on the floor.
(v) Turns about the hands where the hands are placed on the floor, and by springing around them the body can be turned to face the other way.

20

2. Movement by turning

Ask the children to travel across the floor by using turning movements. The turns used can be about the feet or the hands.

Control in landing as well as in the turning movement should be stressed, with landings to be as quiet as possible.

3. Turning without the feet

From a sitting or a lying position the children must turn to face a different direction without using their feet. Ask the children to keep their feet raised throughout this movement. USE MATS.

4. Turning over

Starting the children from a standing or sitting position, ask them how many ways they can find to turn their bodies completely over.

It is possible that cartwheel and forward and backward rolling movements might appear in this activity, if so, the whole class could be given the opportunity to try these. However, if they do not appear naturally in the work such movements should not be introduced. The children will attempt movements such as these when they are ready, which may be at a much later date. USE MATS.

5. Move along the mat

Ask the children to travel along a mat by using turning movements over body parts other than the feet, use of the feet being allowed only where a pupil might start or finish a movement in a standing position.

This activity could be developed by allowing the children to move to each mat in turn and by asking them to travel along each mat using a different turning movement.

6. Standing twists

In a standing position the children try twisting the upper part of their bodies as far as they can to the left and then to the right. The children must try to keep their balance throughout this movement.

7. Corkscrew twists

In a standing position the children first twist the upper part of their bodies to the left, or the right and then follow it with the lower half so that the whole body turns to face a new direction. Ask the children to try turning all the way around by using a succession of corkscrew twists.

This activity can be repeated with the lower half of the body leading the movement and then, in a crouched position, with the children walking their hands around themselves on the floor to see how far they can twist the upper body before the feet have to follow.

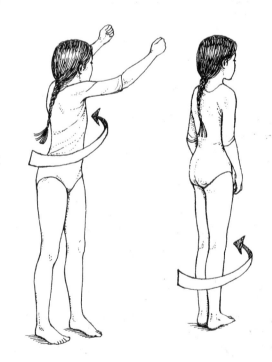

8. Twist to turn

This activity serves to develop the idea of twisting to bring about a turn of the whole body, by allowing the children to explore ways of twisting different body parts in order to initiate a turn. The children can stand or lie down to do this and, by way of stimulating their thoughts, could all begin by lying on their backs to try twisting first their legs and then their upper bodies in order to turn over onto their fronts. When they have done this successfully, ask the children how many ways they can find to twist different body parts in order to get them from their backs onto their fronts and then to try other, different types of body turn. USE MATS.

9. Twist to support

In this activity the children are not particularly required to turn, but rather to transfer their weight through a twisting movement from one body area to another.

From a position of their own choosing, ask the children to twist their bodies in order to take their weight onto a different body part. If they have problems with this idea, the pupils could all try starting from a crouched position and then twist their upper bodies around, so enabling them to topple onto their backs. From this position of lying on their backs the children could then try twisting their upper bodies again to bring them onto their chests. Alternatively, they could bring their knees up to their chests and by twisting and rolling over one shoulder transfer their weight onto their knees and shins. Interesting and quite complex movements can be developed in this activity. USE MATS.

10. Twist and return

In this activity the children use twisting movements to take them from a starting position into a different position and then back again. This can be tried with just two twisting movements at first, for example a twist from lying on the back to lying on the front and then a twist back again. The activity can then be extended into a short sequence where the children have to move through three different positions and then try to return. USE MATS.

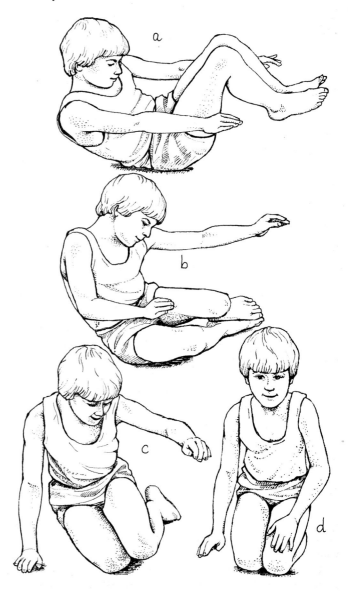

Twist to support.

Main theme: apparatus work

SUITABLE APPARATUS: All forms of apparatus can be used within this theme. Where possible, apparatus such as benches and balancing planks should be raised well off the floor as children are quite adept in twisting and turning around all types of apparatus.

The following activities can be used to develop ideas for both turning and twisting movements. Older pupils might first try the activities using turning movements and then with twisting movements, but for younger pupils who are not able to distinguish between the two, either form of movement can be used.

Emphasis in all the activities should be on balance, control and smoothness in the movements.

1. Turn on and around

Discuss with the class the distinction between the terms 'on' and 'around', perhaps using pieces of apparatus to clarify the difference. A beam is a good piece of apparatus to illustrate this, a child can stand on a beam and make a simple standing turn and then standing on the floor can turn his body over and around the beam in a rolling manner. Having drawn this distinction, ask the children to find different ways of turning on their apparatus and then different ways of turning around it.

2. Turn and return

In this activity the children select a particular turning movement, either a turn on or a turn around the apparatus. Having performed this, they try to return to their original starting position by performing the same movement in reverse.

The children should repeat this activity several times, each time trying a different form of turning movement.

3. Twist and turn around the apparatus

This activity can take different forms:
(i) The children travel about the floor using turning or twisting movements and perform a twisting or a turning movement on or around each piece of apparatus that they come to.
(ii) To focus the children's attention on how they can use different body parts to create and support twisting and turning movements, they can be asked to perform this exercise without using their feet at all for moving and to use them only when they need to stand up in order to mount apparatus.
(iii) A further variation is to ask the children to select a particular turning or twisting movement and to try performing it on each piece of apparatus in turn. This is particularly useful in helping the pupils to appreciate the nature of the different pieces of apparatus and what is possible on them. It also tests their ingenuity and strength, since each piece of apparatus will make very different demands, even though the same movement is being performed.

4. Twist and turn sequence

Using the floor and a piece of apparatus, the children can be asked to develop a sequence where they move onto, across and around the apparatus, travelling throughout by means of twisting and turning movements only.

Here is a simple three-movement sequence which they could begin with: a twisting movement onto the apparatus, a turning movement on or around it and a further twist to come back onto the floor. This sequence could be extended by asking for further movements, or varied by asking for particular types of turning or twisting movement to be included. For example 'Face the apparatus and twist to bring your back or your bottom onto it, turn using a rolling movement and twist off to stand on the floor to face the apparatus again'.

The activity can be further developed by including ideas from the theme of stretching and curling where

23

the children have to adopt stretched and tucked shapes on the apparatus as part of their sequence. This will encourage the children to think of body shape and so aid their general control in the performance of the movements.

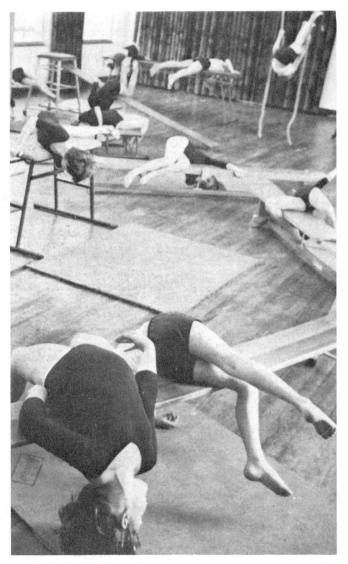

Twisting and turning on apparatus.

Concluding activities

1. Grow and shrink

From a tucked position the children 'grow' slowly by twisting upwards until they are in a fully stretched position. They then have to sink slowly into their original tucked shape. The children must not move their feet and they must try to keep their balance throughout the movement.

2. Snakes

In pairs, one pupil stands with legs apart and the partner, lying face down on the floor, twists in and out of his legs in a figure of eight fashion. The 'snake' must not touch his partner's legs and must also try to keep his feet off the floor throughout the movement.

3. Turn across the floor

The children start on all fours. By moving only two supports at a time, both hands, both feet or one hand and one foot, they have to make their way across the floor using turning movements. They may turn over sideways, using one foot and one hand, bring their feet and their hands alternately round to the front, or they may find a different movement which satisfies the task. The pupils should work in a straight line across the floor. For safety reasons the class may have to work in two halves as each child will occupy a fairly large space when moving.

4. Partner turns

In pairs, the children hold hands and have to move across the floor by turning and without releasing their partner's hands. If mats are left out for this activity the children can try moving down a mat. Interesting variations of movement can appear when mats are made available.

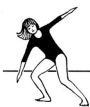 # Movement using other body parts

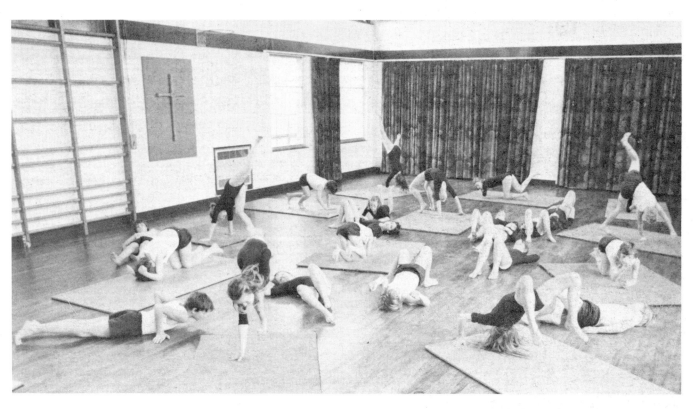

This theme seeks to encourage an awareness of the different ways of propelling the body and to develop imagination and a feel for movement using body areas other than the feet. Much movement on the floor and apparatus relies upon the hands, feet and on rolling activity, but in this theme the children should be encouraged to utilize elbows, knees and heels together with crawling and sliding movements.

The main focus in activities within this theme is on general body control. Use of the feet is to be discouraged and this will mean that the children will be taking their weight on unfamiliar body areas which will create basic balance and control problems.

25

Introductory activities

1. Off the feet 'tag'

This is the same as the normal game of 'tag' where one person has to try and 'tag' the others who then join him in the chase. However, in this activity all movement must be on body parts other than the feet.

2. Tag around a mat

In this activity the children work in pairs with one trying to 'tag' the other around a mat. The children must stay off the mat and also travel on body areas other than the feet. The pupils should take it in turns to do the chasing.

3. Tag around the mats

This is a whole class activity which combines elements of the two previous activities. With the mats spread about the floor, the children have to move around without touching them, travelling on body areas other than the feet. One pupil has to try to 'tag' the others who, if tagged or if they touch a mat, must then join him in the chase.

4. Back to front

The teacher calls out different parts of the body and the children must try to take their weight on just that area. The movement from one body area to the next must be completed by the children without them touching the floor with their feet. Start by calling just 'Back' and 'Front' and then introduce other body areas such as shoulders, side, knees, tummy and bottom.

Main theme: floorwork

1. No feet, no hands

Ask the children to find different ways of travelling about the floor without using their feet or their hands to help them move. The whole class could try some of the more original ideas to emerge.

Encourage slow, controlled movement in the activity.

2. Push and pull

In this activity both feet and hands can be used with the task being for the children to find different ways of travelling about the room using pushing and pulling movements and with the movement being on as many different body areas as they can find. As in the previous activity, the whole class could try some of the more unusual methods to appear.

3. Large areas

This activity and the one which follows (No. 4) introduce the notion of 'large' and 'small' body areas. Once introduced, these terms can be used in all future work where the children must select for themselves the body areas to work on. Being unspecific, the terms in no way influence the form of movement or body parts selected by the children.

In the themes concerned with balance the term 'points' is used when referring to small body areas such as the hands, toes or feet, elbows, knees and head and it would be suitable to use this term in the following activities when working with upper junior classes.

Ask the children to take their weight on a large body area. On the signal, 'Change' they must move onto a different large body area. This movement should be direct and without the use of the hands or the feet.

The children should be able to find at least four large areas to move to, these could include the back, tummy, side, shoulders or upper back, bottom, and shins. By calling, 'Change' and so directing the children's movements, the teacher can stress control and smoothness in the transfer.

After working on this activity in a space or on a mat, the children could try moving across the floor by transferring their weight from one large body area to another.

4. Small areas

This activity is the same as the previous one, but the children are asked to use small body areas. Use of the hands and feet in transferring or in bearing weight should be minimal, and the children should be encouraged to use other small body areas or to use the hands and feet in conjunction with other parts.

Having practised different ways of supporting themselves on small body areas, the children can try moving along by transferring their weight from one small body area to another. USE MATS.

5. Large and small

Using ideas they have obtained from the previous activities, the children can find positions where they are supported alternately on large and small body areas. To stress control in the activity, the movements should be directed by the teacher giving a signal to change position. USE MATS.

This activity can be developed into a movement sequence where the children are asked to travel across the mat, four times, to move alternately on large and small body areas and to make minimal use of the feet and hands.

Main theme: apparatus work

SUITABLE APPARATUS: With the exception of ropes, all apparatus is suitable for work in this theme.

Whilst the object of work in this theme is to discourage the pupil's reliance upon the hands and feet for moving, use of the hands may prove necessary in mounting or in maintaining control on certain pieces of apparatus. The children should be made aware of this and told to use their hands and feet if they feel a real need to.

The children's attention should be focused upon control in all the activities in this section and upon the distinction between large and small body areas. The pupils should also be encouraged to think of body shape and to adopt stretched and curled shapes in their movements as this will benefit their general movement control.

1. On, off and under

This activity can take different forms:
(i) Standing next to a piece of apparatus the children can explore ways of moving onto it and off again without using their feet on the apparatus.

Where the apparatus allows, movement underneath can be tried. Children find interesting and quite unusual ways of using apparatus such as platforms and boxes which allow movement underneath or through the supporting framework. In allowing or encouraging such movements, ensure that the apparatus is stable and not likely to fall. Most free standing apparatus is designed for movement over the top but a child's natural inclination is to move through and under all types of apparatus that allow it.
(ii) The children could try moving onto the apparatus using only large body areas and then only small body areas to transfer their weight.
(iii) Starting from a sitting or a lying position next to the apparatus, the children try to find different

27

ways of moving onto it and returning again to the same position. This variation may only be possible on the lower pieces of apparatus.

2. Across the apparatus

In this activity the children find ways of moving from one side of the apparatus, across it to the other side, without using their feet on the apparatus and using their hands for only minimal control.

As in the previous activity, the children could be asked to use large and small body areas in turn and to try starting from a position off the feet.

With the longer pieces of apparatus, such as benches, the children could be asked to try moving from one end to the other rather than across.

3. Around the apparatus

In this activity the children move to each piece of apparatus in turn, travelling across the floor on body parts other than their feet and hands. At each piece that they come to the children must find a different body part on which to travel along, across or over the apparatus. Throughout the activity the feet and hands should be used only for pushing or pulling and to assist with control on the apparatus. Emphasis in the work should be on the need for smooth and continuous movement.

4. Sequences

For this activity each pupil should work initially on a single piece of apparatus and in the floor space around it. The task for the children is to develop a sequence of three movements where they travel across the floor and onto the apparatus, along it or across it, off again and back across the floor to the starting point, with each of these three movements being on different body areas and with use of the hands and feet being kept to a minimum.

Developments could include further movements or a second piece of apparatus.

Concluding activities

1. Commando crawl

Using benches, both inclined and level, and mats set about the floor, establish a route which the children must follow as 'commandos'. In this they must not stand up at all and must crawl over and under obstacles and up and down the slopes. The mats can be treated as areas of water which the children must cross on their backs with their arms held high as if carrying weapons.

2. Under and out

Arrange the class into small groups, three or four in each group. Each group then stands in a line, one behind the other, facing down the room. On a signal from the teacher the back marker drops to his hands and knees and crawls between the legs of the others in his group to the front. Each back marker in turn does this until the groups reach the other end of the room.

Several variations can be introduced:
(i) Face the pupils the other way so that all movement is backwards.
(iii) Ask the pupils to go through the tunnel on their backs and then on their tummies.
(iii) Ask them to form the tunnel from different body shapes, such as bridges on the hands and feet.

3. Wriggle about and out

This activity is similar to the previous one, but here the pupils sit in a line with their legs tucked in and with a gap between each team member. On a signal from the teacher the back marker, lying on his back, has to wriggle and weave in and out of the rest of the team to the front of the line. Each back marker has to do this in turn until all team members have been through once.

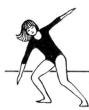

Rolling

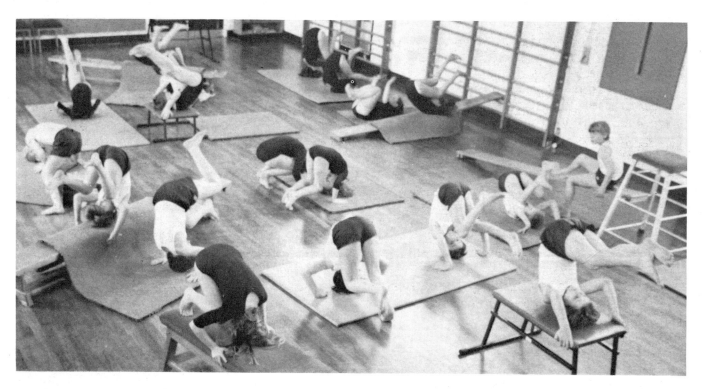

Work in this theme greatly assists a child's development of body and spatial awareness. It involves rotational work, which takes the child through inverted positions, and travelling movements where he needs to be certain of a clear path before setting off. The ability to perform rolls with confidence also provides the child with a safe escape route in work where bad landings might occur and, in a more positive sense, is the forerunner of many of the more advanced skills met in gymnastics.

Introductory activities

1. Mat roll

Space all the mats around the floor with the children sitting in the remaining floor space. On a signal from the teacher the children run and cross every mat using a rolling movement and then return to their original place. To avoid the possibility of collisions make it a rule that only one person may cross a mat at a time or that rolls must be performed lengthways on the mats. A further safety precaution is to have only half of the class working at a time; this also allows the pupils to work more quickly and far more vigorously.

2. Mat roll chase

For this activity the children work in pairs on a single mat. If there are insufficient mats the children could be grouped in threes with each pupil taking a turn to sit out.

The pupils begin the activity standing on opposite sides of their mat. On a signal from the teacher, one pupil rolls across the mat whilst the other runs around the end. Both pupils then follow this same route of rolling across the mat and running around the end in an effort to catch up and 'tag' their partner. The mat must only be crossed in one direction using a rolling movement and must not be touched by the pupils as they run around the end. A pupil can only 'tag' his partner from behind.

A maximum of ten seconds should be allowed for this activity before a halt is called and the children given a rest.

3. Step over, roll under

The pupils again work in pairs on a single mat.

In this activity the children cross the mat in one direction by using a sideways rolling movement and in the opposite direction by stepping or jumping over the mat. By starting on opposite sides of the mat the pupils can work together, with the stepping movement being over both the partner and the mat.

The more accomplished pupils might wish to try using tucked forward or backward rolls to cross the mat, with the partner using a straddle or leapfrog shape in jumping over.

Main theme: floorwork

Mats will be necessary for all the activities in this section.

It is appropriate in this theme to teach the techniques for controlled forward and backward rolls. These are quite specific movement skills which, once mastered, considerably broaden a child's scope for developing movement ideas in all the themes of work. The teacher may need to support or steady the movement of some children in these activities.

1. Different rolls

Ask the pupils to find different ways of rolling across a mat.

A wide variety of ideas will emerge which all the children could try and which can be developed by focusing upon different aspects of the movements:
(i) Shape: Ask the children to roll in both stretched and tucked shapes and highlight the different points of style; body fully extended or body tightly tucked in.
(ii) Direction: Ask the children to roll in forward, backward and sideways directions.
(iii) Use of the hands: Some children may use their hands to help them in rolling, others may not. This difference in technique, if apparent, can be explored by the whole class.

In all of this work, the need for control in the movements and concentration on shape throughout the rolling phase needs to be stressed. A tucked roll should stay tightly tucked and the body should remain fully extended throughout a stretched rolling movement.

2. The backward roll

This skill can be developed most easily by taking the children through a series of movements which lead up to the full roll.

(**i**) The pupils start in a tightly crouched position with the backs of their hands on their shoulders.

(**ii**) From this position they topple backwards off their feet, rolling from their bottoms onto their backs and shoulders and reaching to put the palms of their hands on the floor.

(**iii**) This movement is repeated with the children reaching for the floor with each foot in turn. This action will direct the rolling movement over each shoulder and the children should try to take their body weight on the toes of the leading foot, first over the left shoulder and then over the right.

(**iv**) Having practised the previous activity at length, the children should be encouraged to quicken up the movement and to try to straighten up the direction of the roll. When they can do this, the body weight can be taken over both hands and onto the feet. Encourage the children to roll quickly, to stay tucked up tightly throughout the movement, and to curl up the toes in readiness to receive the body weight on the feet.

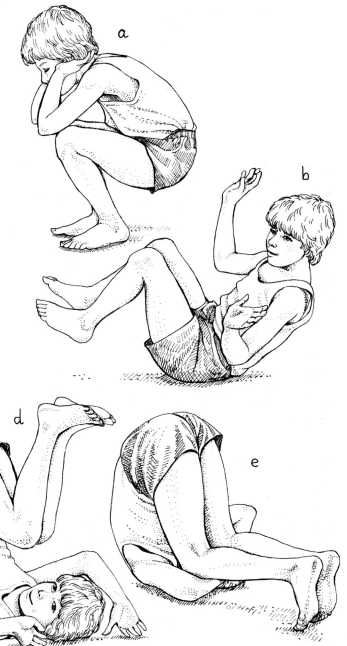

3. The forward roll

As soft a work surface as possible should be provided for those children who experience real difficulties with this movement.

As with the backward roll, this movement should be built up through a series of stages.

(**i**) The pupils start from a crouched position with their heads tucked in tightly between their knees.

(**ii**) Placing their hands on the floor close to their feet the children topple forwards and sideways over one shoulder. Emphasize that the hands must be placed firmly on the floor as many children have a tendency to turn the hand and tuck the leading arm under their body when rolling over their shoulders.

(**iii**) This movement can be repeated many times with the children passing over each shoulder in turn.

(**iv**) When this movement is being performed confidently the children should be encouraged to spring slightly into the roll, rather than just toppling forward, and to try to roll straight. The children must keep their heads in and stay tightly tucked, like a ball, until their body weight moves onto their feet.

The head should never touch the mat in this movement and a slight spring from the feet allows the head to be tucked under so that the shoulders make first contact on the mat.

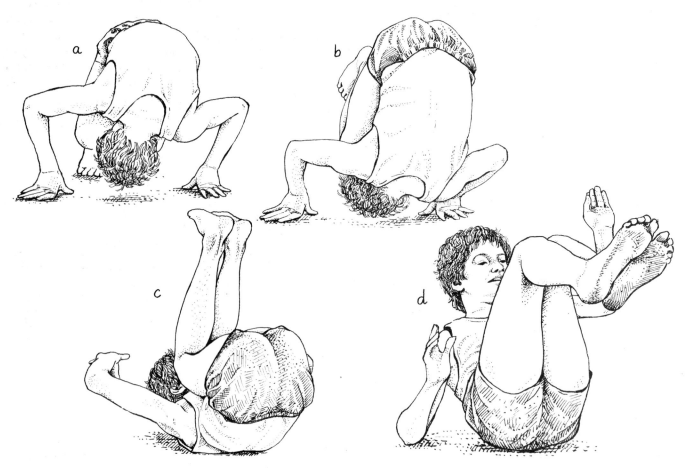

4. Starts and finishes

The rolling movements explored in the previous activities can all be developed by focusing upon starting and finishing positions.

(i) Starts: Ask the children to choose one of the rolling movements they have enjoyed working on and to try performing it from different starting positions. These could include crouching, standing, a straddle stance with legs apart, or a lying position.

(ii) Finishes: The same procedure can then be used with the focus being on different finishing positions. Ask the children to try finishing their roll in a crouched position, then by coming upright onto their feet, then in a straddle position, and then to try to find other controlled finishing positions.

5. Floor sequence

Ask the children to develop a sequence of three rolls across a mat, starting and finishing in a standing position.

This activity can be extended by developing all the different parts of the sequence, the rolling movements and the start and finishing positions. The children could be asked to include particular types of rolling movement in their sequence, for example a forward roll or a sideways stretched roll. They could be asked to include rolls in particular directions, perhaps along as well as across the mat. Starts and finishes could be crouched, upright or in a straddle position. Once the children have explored all these various possibilities in their sequence it could then be further developed by introducing extra rolls.

In this activity the emphasis needs to be on control of movement. Each part of the children's sequences should have a definite start and finish and one roll ought not to lead straight into the next.

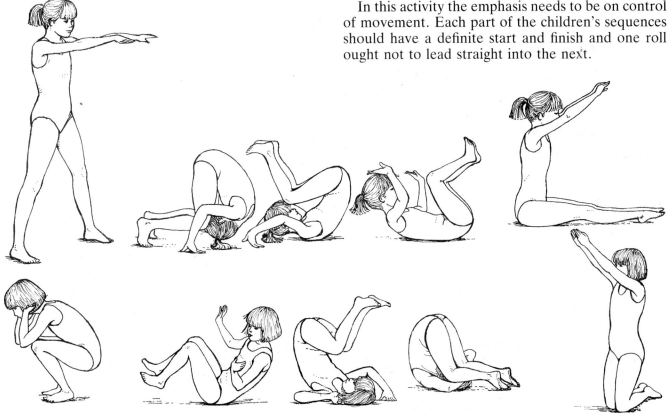

33

Main theme: apparatus work

SUITABLE APPARATUS: All forms of flat-topped apparatus can be used, with the ideal arrangement offering work surfaces of different widths and heights and also surfaces which are slightly inclined. All the surfaces should be sufficiently low that the children can use rolling movements to get onto and off the apparatus and be sufficiently wide that the children can work with confidence. All the apparatus needs to be padded and additional soft surfaces can be made by draping agility mats over benches and balancing planks.

1. Roll on, roll aìong

The children stand on the floor against a piece of apparatus and find different ways of moving onto it using rolling movements. They can then stand, sit or lie on the apparatus and find different ways of rolling along it.

This activity can be developed by asking the children to try particular types of rolling movement or by asking them to start and finish a movement in a particular position, for example with feet together, or standing up.

The main points to emphasize in this activity are the selection of rolling movements that are appropriate to a piece of apparatus, control in rolling to ensure that the movement stays on the apparatus, and the maintenance of shape throughout the movement.

2. Over and across

In this activity the children find different ways of rolling across the apparatus, from the floor on one side to the floor on the other. It is essential that a soft landing surface is provided, as the children may have difficulty in controlling their movements in the early attempts.

Rolling movements across apparatus tend to be much quicker than when the same rolls are performed along the apparatus. The children should therefore be asked to try to hold their finishing position, this will have the effect of slowing the movement down and help the children with their overall control.

3. Roll around the apparatus

In this activity the children move to each piece of apparatus in turn and travel over, across or along it using a rolling movement. Aspects of work from other themes can be included in the activity, for example the children can be asked to travel between the apparatus on body parts other than the feet.

As a variation, the children could be asked to choose one rolling movement and to try performing it on each of the pieces of apparatus. They would find this to be quite a challenging exercise as the movement would have to be continually modified to satisfy the particular nature of each piece of apparatus.

4. Develop a sequence

The children could base their work in this activity around a single piece of apparatus or a limited arrangement of two or three pieces, this will depend upon the age and the ability of the children. Younger children may find it easier to work with the variety of alternatives presented by several different pieces of apparatus, whilst it might be more beneficial to the development of movement skill in the older pupils if they have to confine their routine to just a single piece of apparatus and the floor space which surrounds it.

Ask the children to develop a sequence of just four rolling movements at first, with two rolls being on the apparatus and two on the floor. As the children become proficient in performing this sequence the number of movements can be increased or they can be asked to include movements and shapes of particular kinds.

The focus in this activity should be on control, with each movement in the sequence having a definite start and finish.

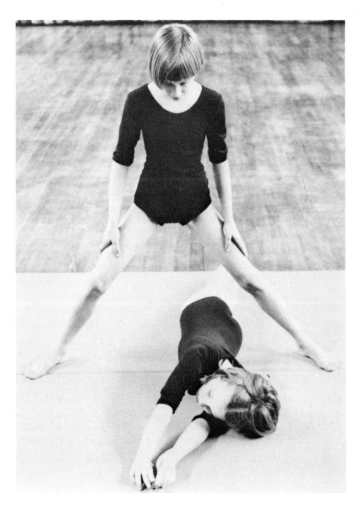

Two pupils in starting positions for the activity 'Roll me down'.

Concluding activities

1. Roll me down

Working in pairs, one pupil lies stretched whilst the partner stands astride him. On a signal from the teacher, the pupil who is lying down has to roll sideways, to and fro, in an attempt to touch his partner's legs with his body. At the same time, the standing partner has to move quickly to the left and the right in order to keep his legs away and so prevent this from happening. A set time of perhaps ten seconds should be allowed, after which the pupils should change places. USE MATS.

2. Criss-cross rolls

Once children have developed reasonable control and confidence in performing rolling movements, they will enjoy working with another pupil on partner routines. A simple activity of this type is where one pupil rolls down a mat and the partner rolls across it and they work alternately in a criss-cross fashion. The pupils can work on the routine to improve their timing, whereby their bodies pass more closely and also travel quicker. They can also introduce return movements of a different kind so that they each cross and re-cross the mat using two different rolls.

3. Over and under

A more ambitious partner routine is where one pupil rolls along a mat and the partner performs a roll, usually a forward roll, over the top.

This activity should be used with the more able gymnasts as it can lead to quite interesting and adventurous movements if the pupil who passes underneath tries different types of roll.

35

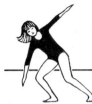

Movement using the hands

The ability to take one's weight on the hands is very important in gymnastics as it opens up a whole new range of movement possibilities. It benefits a child's spatial and body awareness by allowing him to move into inverted positions and generally contributes to control in several of the other movement themes.

Partner support work, as an aid to developing movement on the hands, should not be introduced until the children are at least able to support their own weight. Some pupils may be unable to take their weight on their hands for more than the briefest moment and if held up by someone could collapse and sustain injury. Support work is something which needs to be taught very carefully as incorrect supporting can result in injury to both the supporter and the gymnast.

Introductory activities

1. Bunny-hop races

The children crouch down on one side of the room and on a signal from the teacher must cross the floor and return using the bunny-hop technique for moving. In this, the children reach forward on the floor with their hands and then bring their feet up to their hands with a little spring.

Variations on this activity can include 'bunny-hop tag', where the children play a normal game of 'tag' but have to move using the bunny-hop technique, and 'bunny-hop chase' in which the children work in pairs with one pupil chasing the other around the floor or around a mat.

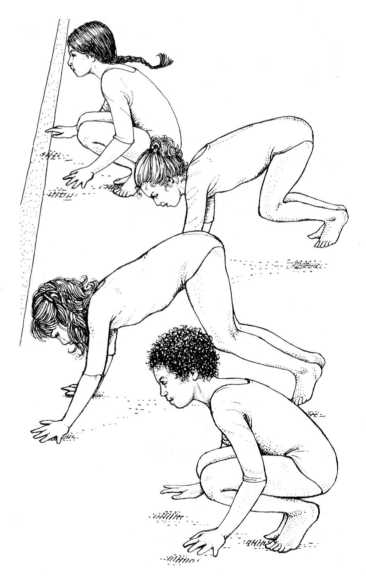

2. Spider races

This activity is similar to the previous one, with the same variations being possible. However, movement in this activity is on all fours, and the children keep their arms and legs straight. In this position, they can move fairly quickly by bringing their legs around the sides of their body.

Both this and bunny-hopping are difficult movements to perform backwards and the children will have fun trying to race backwards across the floor.

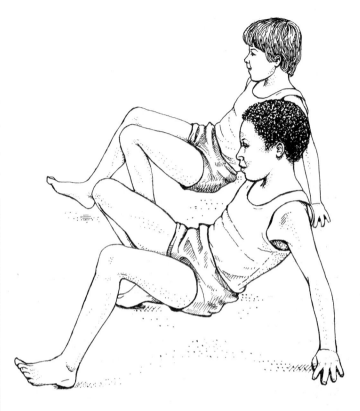

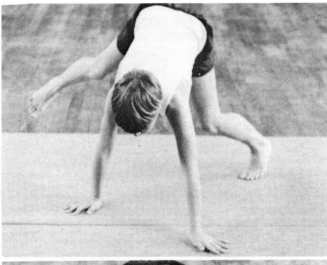

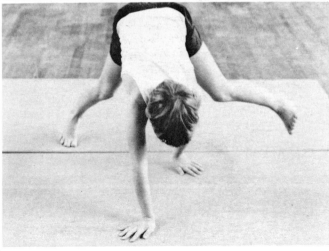

3. Crab races

This activity again follows the format used in 'bunny-hop races' but the children support themselves on all fours with their bottoms towards the floor.

4. Partner tag on a mat

The children work in pairs with one mat to each pair.

Supporting themselves on all fours with hands on the mat and feet on the floor and starting on opposite sides of the mat, one pupil has to try to 'tag' his partner. Both pupils must keep their hands on the mat and feet on the floor throughout the chase and when the chaser eventually 'tags' his partner, the two of them can change roles and start again. Movement can be in any direction.

Main theme: floorwork

Floorwork in this theme focuses upon two broad areas, the 'support' function of the hands and the 'transfer of weight' function. In the first, there is little movement of the body across the floor, the arms support the body weight longer and are responsible for much of the control in the movement. In the second, the body moves over the hands, hand contact with the floor is for a much shorter time, and movement, which tends to be fairly quick, is initiated by the feet; the function of the hands is to merely transfer this movement across the floor.

1. Onto and off the hands

This activity can take several different forms:
(i) From a crouched position, with their hands on the floor, the children spring up onto their hands and land again on the same spot. Their hands should be placed shoulder width apart on the floor, arms should be kept straight and the legs tucked up. This activity could be likened to a bunny-hop on the spot, with the bottom lifted high in the movement. Ask the children to see how long they can keep their feet off the floor, this encourages balance control and indicates arm strength and the children's general level of readiness for work which lays stress on the support function of the hands.

The variations which follow will help the children to develop ideas for moving on the hands.
(ii) Moving forwards: From a crouched position the children spring forward onto their hands and bring their feet up to follow. The emphasis in this movement should be on the spring onto the hands. Unlike a bunny-hop, where the hands can slide forward across the floor, this movement should be one where the hands take far more weight with the body momentarily landing on the hands.
(iii) Moving backwards: In this the children spring onto their hands but then push away so that the feet move backwards.

(iv) Turning: The children spring onto their hands and turn in the air so that a quarter turn has been completed when the feet land. This same movement can be achieved by placing the hands down with a quarter turn, so that the body then straightens out in the jumping action. The children should try to make turns to both the left and the right, keep their legs together throughout the movement and try to land without losing balance.

2. Weight transfer

Ask the children to find different ways of moving over a mat, first by placing both hands on the mat and then by using only one hand.

The emphasis in this activity should be on control, both of the movement and the landing, and body shape. The children should try to use stretched or tucked shapes in travelling across their mats as this will enhance the appearance of the movement and help them in maintaining control.

3. Hands and roll sequence

Ask the children to develop a sequence where they move across a mat three times, first with the hands only touching the mat, then with a roll and then again by using the hands.

The use of two forms of movement in the sequence will help the children to appreciate how movements of quite different kinds can be combined in the development of simple routines. The emphasis in this activity should be on control, with the children trying to complete each movement on their feet.

Main theme: apparatus work

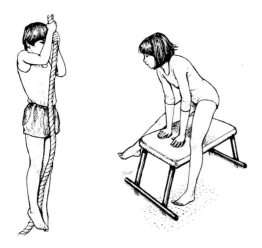

SUITABLE APPARATUS: Climbing frame, beams, upright and upturned benches, ropes and low platforms.

Body weight can be taken by the hands above as well as below the body in this theme. This should be pointed out to the children and they can be encouraged to try movements in hanging positions.

1. On and off

Working on a single piece of apparatus, the children find different ways of getting onto and off their particular piece by using only their hands and their feet. The children must try to avoid touching the apparatus with any other part of their body.

2. Hands on, hands off

In this activity the children move onto the apparatus by taking their weight on their hands. For example, the hands can be placed on the apparatus and the rest of the body brought on by jumping up. On very low apparatus, such as benches, the more confident pupil might get on by using a cartwheel type of movement. On apparatus such as ropes and beams, where hanging positions are possible, the children might try pulling themselves up by their hands.

Having got onto the apparatus, the children's movements to get off must also be supported by the hands. *The children must not be allowed to try jumping down onto their hands.* The hands should either be placed on the apparatus and be the last part of the body to leave it, or they should be placed firmly on the floor to support the movement.

Having worked on a single piece of apparatus, the children should be given the opportunity to try the activity on other pieces. This will help them to appreciate the different types of apparatus.

3. Hands over and across

In this activity the children have to try moving over the apparatus by touching it only with their hands. If ropes, wallbars or climbing frames are part of the apparatus arrangement, the instruction should be to move onto and off them or across them by using hands only.

The children's attention should be focused upon control in take-off and landing and on body shape during the movement phase. The children should try to travel in tucked or stretched positions as the legs can be very untidy in this movement and concentrating upon maintaining a particular shape has a considerable effect upon overall control.

4. Sequence on the floor and apparatus

Using one piece of apparatus and the floor space around it, the children can try to develop a sequence of four movements where they travel with their weight supported principally by the hands. The sequence should include two movements on the floor and two on the apparatus.

Younger pupils could be asked to find just three movements, with the task being to move across the floor, across the apparatus and then back across the floor with body weight being supported at all times on just the hands and feet.

Concluding activities

1. Crab football

To play this game the children support themselves on all fours, as described in the 'crab races' activity. The children can move anywhere but must do so by walking on their hands and feet and not by sliding on their bottoms. One or two large, lightweight balls are required, and the class needs to be organized into two teams. Each team defends one end wall of the room and tries to score by kicking or heading the ball against the opposite wall. The ball must not be played with the hands. Using two balls at the same time adds considerably to the fun and also to the number of goals scored.

2. Cartwheel and bridge walk

Two of the more formal gymnastic movements which could be introduced to the children as a concluding activity to a lesson are the cartwheel and the bridge support position.

In performing a cartwheel the children should endeavour to travel in a straight line and try to keep their arms and legs as straight as possible throughout the movement.

All pupils should be encouraged to practise the bridge support position as it is so valuable in helping to maintain flexibility in the shoulder joints. The position can take two forms and in either of these the children can try to walk forwards and backwards and they can even have short races if the skill is particularly well developed.

Two bridge support positions.

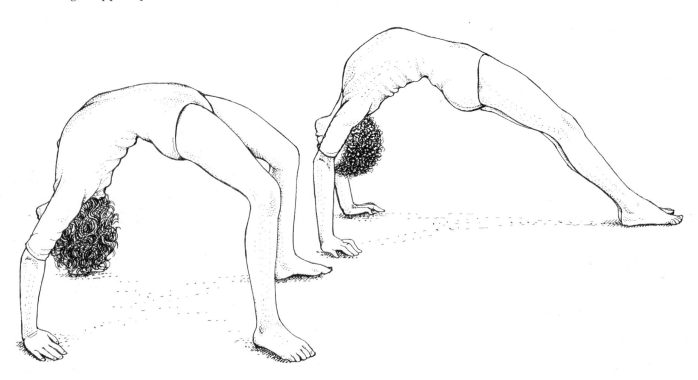

40

Take-off and landing

The skills of take-off and landing are important in many areas of gymnastics, and particularly so in work involving apparatus. It is therefore essential that children recognize these as distinct areas of movement skill and be given the opportunity to develop them in their own right within a gymnastics programme.

Take-off and landing skills are of particular significance to movements concerned with flight and consideration of the principles connected with these skills can form a useful introduction to lessons in the flight themes.

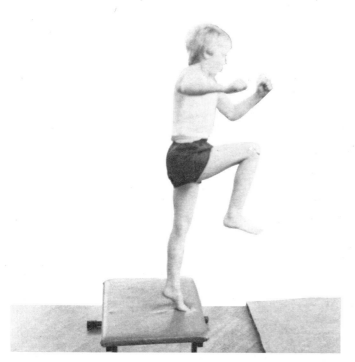

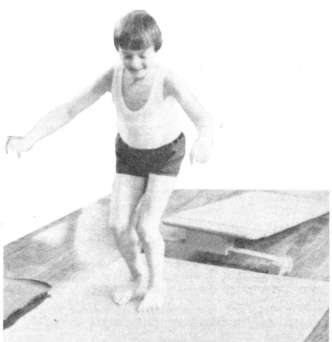

Introductory activities

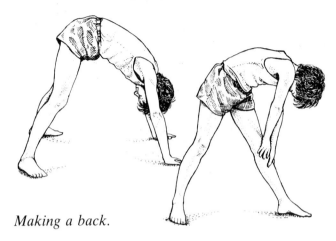

Making a back.

1. Leap-frog

Organize the class into pairs, ensuring that the children are with someone of a similar height and build. The activity can then take several forms:

(i) Leap-frogging on the move: where a pair leap-frog alternately and progress across the floor. The class should work from side to side across the room.

(ii) Static leap-frog: where each pupil in turn performs a given number of leaps over his partner. This could take the form of a race where each partner has to complete five leaps and the teacher looks for the first pair to finish.

(iii) Over and under: where each pupil in turn completes a given number of movements, perhaps five, leap-frogging over his partner's back and returning under his legs.

It is important in this activity to instruct the children on how to stand when 'making a back' for someone to leap-frog over. Legs and arms should be straight and the back firm. If this is not the case, the person making the back can collapse and the person who is leap-frogging may land awkwardly.

With very young children a safe and effective 'back' can be made by tucking up tightly on the knees.

2. Run and jump

The children run around the floor into spaces and when the teacher claps hands they have to jump as high as possible and try to hold their landing position, moving off again when the teacher gives the command 'Run'.

Main theme: floorwork

1. Standing jump take-off

Ask the children to jump as high as they can from a standing position. When the children have repeated this several times, ask them to try jumping off just one leg and to drive the other leg upwards in the jump. The children can then try both types to decide if either gives them greater height.

2. Running jump take-off

If there is little space available this activity is best performed with the children all working across the floor and jumping in the same direction.

Ask the children to run and spring as high as possible into the air. When they have tried this several times, ask them to try both a one-footed and a two-footed take-off from a run and to note which feels the more natural and which seems to give the greatest height.

3. Standing versus running

In this activity the children compare the height gained from standing and running jumps. This can be done with the class working in pairs and with each pair using a stretch of clear wall on which to measure their jumping height.

The first jump should be from standing, with the pupils standing sideways to the wall and jumping to touch it as high as possible with the nearest hand.

They can
touch it, a
at about t
   Conside
can includ
athletics,
from one
catch a ba
with a on

4. Jump

The two
with an er
parts of t
height in a
the swing
use of the
also be dr

5. Quiet

Any of t
repeated,
their jump
what they
and if the
activity, fi
as quietly

6. Whoc

This activ
landing.
   Ask the
by leaning
swinging th
balance or
older pupi
technique
identify fo
to be cons

Introductory activities

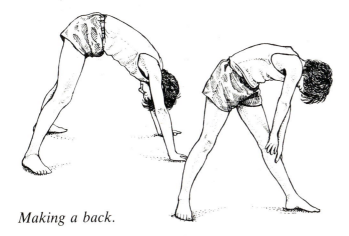

Making a back.

1. Leap-frog

Organize the class into pairs, ensuring that the children are with someone of a similar height and build. The activity can then take several forms:
(i) Leap-frogging on the move: where a pair leap-frog alternately and progress across the floor. The class should work from side to side across the room.
(ii) Static leap-frog: where each pupil in turn performs a given number of leaps over his partner. This could take the form of a race where each partner has to complete five leaps and the teacher looks for the first pair to finish.
(iii) Over and under: where each pupil in turn completes a given number of movements, perhaps five, leap-frogging over his partner's back and returning under his legs.
   It is important in this activity to instruct the children on how to stand when 'making a back' for someone to leap-frog over. Legs and arms should be straight and the back firm. If this is not the case, the person making the back can collapse and the person who is leap-frogging may land awkwardly.
   With very young children a safe and effective 'back' can be made by tucking up tightly on the knees.

2. Run and jump

The children run around the floor into spaces and when the teacher claps hands they have to jump as high as possible and try to hold their landing position, moving off again when the teacher gives the command 'Run'.

Main theme: floorwork

1. Standing jump take-off

Ask the children to jump as high as they can from a standing position. When the children have repeated this several times, ask them to try jumping off just one leg and to drive the other leg upwards in the jump. The children can then try both types to decide if either gives them greater height.

2. Running jump take-off

If there is little space available this activity is best performed with the children all working across the floor and jumping in the same direction.
   Ask the children to run and spring as high as possible into the air. When they have tried this several times, ask them to try both a one-footed and a two-footed take-off from a run and to note which feels the more natural and which seems to give the greatest height.

3. Standing versus running

In this activity the children compare the height gained from standing and running jumps. This can be done with the class working in pairs and with each pair using a stretch of clear wall on which to measure their jumping height.
   The first jump should be from standing, with the pupils standing sideways to the wall and jumping to touch it as high as possible with the nearest hand.

They can then run alongside the wall to jump and touch it, again with the nearest hand and preferably at about the same spot, to facilitate comparison.

Consideration of the merits of each type of jump can include discussion on high jumping technique in athletics, where the athletes always run and take off from one foot, and jumping against someone to catch a ball, which is also best done from a run and with a one-footed take-off.

4. Jumping aids

The two previous activities can both be repeated with an emphasis being placed on how the different parts of the body can contribute towards gaining height in a jump. Attention should be focused upon the swing of the arms upwards to give lift and the use of the 'free leg' in a running jump which can also be driven upwards at take-off.

5. Quiet landings

Any of the previous take-off activities can be repeated, with the children being asked to land from their jump as quietly as possible. Ask the children what they do to reduce the noise of their landing and if they seem uncertain let them repeat the activity, first landing as noisily as possible and then as quietly as possible.

6. Whoops!

This activity focuses attention upon control in landing.

Ask the children to perform standing jumps and by leaning their bodies, tilting their heads or swinging their arms about to see if they can influence balance on landing. When using this activity with older pupils, a discussion should follow on the best technique for landing. Older juniors will usually identify for themselves all the elements which need to be considered.

The correct landing position should be with the toes and balls of the feet meeting the floor first. Ankles and knees should be bent to cushion the force and the whole body should sink slightly. The head and upper body should be kept straight and should lean forward slightly in order to avoid falling backwards and the arms should be held out to the side to help maintain balance.

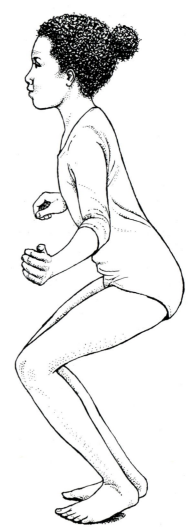

Correct position for landing.

7. Running jump to land

This activity is best performed with the children working in the same direction across the floor.

Ask the children to run quickly, to jump and to control their landing as well as possible. Landing from a running jump usually involves the use of an extra step, with the front leg acting as a brake. The need for this extra step will probably be immediately apparent, although the younger children may have to be shown how the leg reaches forward and bends at the knee in order to cushion the forward movement. Older pupils should be allowed to experiment with this jumping movement in order to decide for themselves how the front leg acts to control the landing.

8. One-footed landing

This is a difficult exercise but one which will benefit the children's balance and general control in landing.

Ask the children to try landing on one foot from both standing and running jumps. The emphasis should be on control and the part played by the arms and the 'free leg' in maintaining balance.

Main theme: apparatus work

SUITABLE APPARATUS: Springboards, benches and very low platforms for jumping off, mats for jumping onto and over.

The intention within this section of the work is to focus the children's attention even more closely upon control in take-off and landing by presenting them with situations which demand a little more accuracy in both of these areas. It is essential that the children do not feel apprehensive about performing take-off and landing movements on the apparatus and for this reason very low apparatus should be used. Concern with flight and aspects of movement which require more time in the air, and therefore higher apparatus, are dealt with in other themes.

1. Land on

Ask the children to run and spring onto a piece of apparatus and to try to make a controlled landing on two feet. Younger pupils should each work on a single piece of apparatus and move to another piece on the teacher's direction. Older pupils can progress from piece to piece around the apparatus but to avoid collisions and congestion a route should be decided upon for moving around it, or there should be an understanding as to which direction each piece of apparatus is to be approached from.

2. Jump off

Using just the benches and platforms the children stand on a piece of apparatus and make a two-footed jump to land on a mat. Quietness and control in landing should be stressed and the points made in the floorwork on how these qualities can be achieved could be revised. The children will quickly realize that the extra height gained in jumping off apparatus makes increased demands upon their ability to control a landing, and they should be encouraged to jump both forwards and backwards in order to develop this skill.

3. Jump over

This is a further activity to develop landing skill in which the children must try to jump over a mat to make a controlled two-footed landing on the other side. If the mats are large and difficult to jump over then the children can jump across a corner instead.

Because of the speed involved in this movement the children should be encouraged to use an extra step on landing if they cannot achieve immediate control on two feet.

4. Running jump from the apparatus

Springboards, benches and balancing planks on the floor or suspended very low can be used.

Ask the children to run and take off from the apparatus with two feet and to make a controlled two-footed landing on a mat.

Some children have considerable difficulty with this activity in synchronising their running and adjusting their step to meet the take-off point with their feet together. Where this occurs, the pupils should approach the take-off with just a one-step lead-in and gradually increase the number of steps and then the speed from walking to running.

5. Safety roll

It is extremely beneficial if children can learn how to escape safely from bad landings as injuries do sometimes occur where children land badly, over-balance and instinctively reach out with their hands to break their fall. The main point to stress to the children with regard to bad landings is that the hands should not be stretched out to break the fall, that the force of the body falling needs to be used up in some way, and that this is best achieved by performing a rolling movement.

Using mats, the children should first revise work done on forward and backward rolls, starting from a crouched position and then rising until they lead into the rolls from a standing position. This can then be followed with the children jumping down from a bench, forwards and then backwards and moving immediately into a roll on landing.

6. Sequences of jumps and landings

Using the floor and a piece of apparatus, the children can develop combinations of jumps involving different take-offs and landings.

As an introduction to later work involving movement in flight the children might also include turning movements in their jumps.

Concluding activities

1. Jumping statues

The children jog about the floor and when the teacher claps hands they jump and try to hold their landing position until the teacher gives the signal to move again.

This activity can be used as an elimination game with pupils who overbalance on landing or who move during the period of stillness being given out.

2. Standing long jump

This activity can take the form of a little competition with the children working in pairs, one against the other.

Use lines marked on the floor, a wall or a bench set on its side as the take-off marker. To perform a jump the children stand with feet together and with heels touching the marker and from this position they spring forward as far as possible. The jump will only count if the landing is controlled, with feet still together. The distance of the jump is marked by the partner at the point where the heels reach.

3. Do as I do

In this activity the children can work in pairs or in groups of three, each group requiring a mat. Taking it in turns to lead the group, one pupil performs a jumping movement of his own choosing to cross the mat. Any type of jump is allowed but the landing must be controlled. The other members of the group must then repeat exactly this jumping movement. If the activity is used as a game, then each pupil can start with five lives, forfeiting one life each time they lose balance and control in a jump. The pupil with most lives at the end of the session is the winner.

If the mats are too wide for younger pupils to jump, they can perform the activity by jumping over one corner.

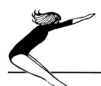 # Shape in flight

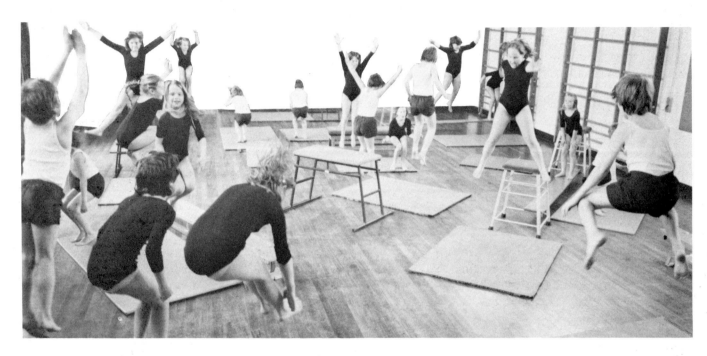

It is important for children to think of flight as a separate phase of movement from the take-off and the landing. Shapes or movements performed in the air should be initiated and completed during the flight phase and they should have little influence upon the other two elements.

The performance of any movement during flight requires time and this time is dependent upon the height achieved in jumping. This should be stressed as a means of encouraging pupils to work for maximum lift in their take-off. The early introduction of apparatus will also benefit the development of ideas and movement skills in this theme as jumps from apparatus give the pupils sufficient time to complete shapes prior to landing, something which they might find difficult when jumping off the floor.

It is essential, for safety reasons, that pupils adopt a correct position when landing. In concentrating on the performance of a shape, pupils can sometimes land whilst coming out of a movement. Sufficient practice should therefore be given in adopting simple shapes in the air in order that each pupil appreciates the time that they are in flight, in this way they will be better able to assess what shapes to attempt in the time available to them.

Introductory activities

As an introduction to work in this theme, the skills involved in take-off and landing should be revised. The activities requiring a two-footed take-off in the previous theme and those focusing attention upon safe, quiet and controlled landing should be included, together with work on rolling out of a bad landing.

For the next two activities, use apparatus as indicated in the apparatus work section, with a mat placed next to each piece.

1. Jump down and roll

The children move around the apparatus, climbing or jumping onto each piece and jumping down with feet together, moving immediately into a roll when their feet touch the mats.

2. Jump and hold

To revise landing technique and to focus the children's attention more upon flight time, before they try to perform movements during the flight phase, the previous activity can be repeated with the children trying to hold their landing positions on the mats.

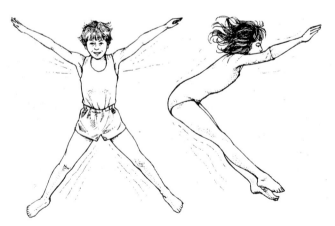

Main theme: floorwork

1. Stretch and tuck

This is a simple activity to remind the children of the two basic shapes they might perform in flight. Ask the children to see how many stretched and how many tucked shapes they can perform when standing on either one or two feet. In performing tucked shapes the pupils should crouch with their knees to their chests but with their heads kept upright as this is the position they will need to assume in flight. If the head is dropped towards the knees when making a tucked shape in the air, the body begins to rotate forwards; a safe and controlled landing then becomes very difficult.

2. Off the floor, off a bench

Ask the children to perform either a tucked shape or a stretched shape in the air, first by jumping off and landing on the floor and then by jumping off a bench and landing on a mat. Older children might discuss what the differences are between the two jumps, with the height and time factors and how they influence performance being considered.

3. Letters in the air

In this activity the children try to perform letter shapes in the air. They could first attempt this by jumping off the floor but the activity should be transferred quite quickly onto the apparatus, this will give the children more time in flight to attempt the different shapes that are possible. Letters which the children might begin with are: I, T, X, C and Y.

Main theme: apparatus work

SUITABLE APPARATUS: Low platforms, benches, springboards and mats. As the children gain in confidence, the height of the apparatus can be slowly increased.

It is essential in all activities involving flight that the children have definite landing areas which must not be crossed. Mats should be positioned next to each piece of apparatus and the instructions given that all movement off apparatus must be onto the mats and that nobody should cross a mat when moving around the apparatus.

1. Around the apparatus

Ask the children to move to each piece of apparatus in turn, to jump off and to perform a stretched or a tucked shape in flight with a controlled two-footed landing on the mat. Allow the children to make standing or running jumps off the apparatus.

As the children show more confidence, higher pieces of apparatus should be introduced.

2. Tuck and stretch sequence

With each pupil working on a piece of apparatus of his own choosing, ask the children to perform three different shapes in flight, to include two stretched shapes and one tucked shape. The three jumps must all be off the apparatus and onto the mat. Ask the children to try keeping their feet together at all times other than when they are performing their shapes in the air; this will help to ensure that correct landing positions are adopted following each jump and also that the children use methods for moving onto the apparatus other than just climbing on.

3. Shape, turn or roll sequence

This activity requires the children to combine the ideas they have developed in this theme with the movement forms of turning and rolling. The children could work around a single piece of apparatus or two or three adjacent pieces.

Ask the children to develop a sequence of three shapes in flight where movement back to or between the apparatus is by rolls or turns. Control in landing and in completing rolls and turns should be stressed, so that the different parts of the sequence can be identified.

Concluding activities

1. O'Grady says

For this activity the children work in a space and perform shapes as directed by the teacher's commands. These shapes may be performed by the children either standing or lying down with the commands including; 'Be wide', 'Be thin', 'Be tucked', 'Be curved'. The activity can take the form of a game with the children having to make the appropriate shape only when the teacher's command is prefaced by the words, 'O'Grady says', and being eliminated if they move when these words are not used.

2. Form a word

Working in pairs the children take it in turns to spell out a word by forming letter shapes in flight with partners trying to guess the word being spelt. Because of the difficulty in forming certain letter shapes, ask the children to use words of only two, three or four letters and allow them to tell their partner one letter of a three-letter word and two letters of a four-letter word. USE BENCHES AND MATS.

48

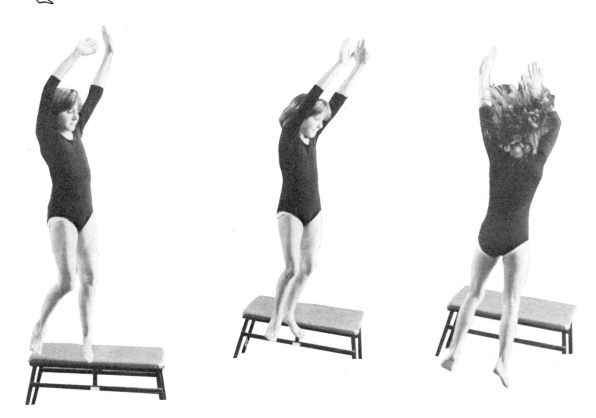

Movement in flight

Three stages of turning 180 degrees in flight.

Work within this theme focuses upon movements which bring about a change in the body's orientation during flight. Height in jumping, which creates time for movement, and twisting and turning actions of the body, which bring about the changes in direction, are elements which are fundamental to successful performance in this work.

Introductory activities

Because of the importance of height in jumping and control in landing, together with the actions of twisting and turning to create movement, floorwork activities taken from the themes of 'Twisting and turning' and 'Take-off and landing' serve as ideal introductory activities for lessons in this theme. Particularly suitable are the activities, 'How can we turn', 'Standing twists', 'Corkscrew twists', 'Standing jump take-off' and 'Running jump take-off'.

Main theme: floorwork

1. Jump with a twist

Turns can be initiated in the jumping action by coiling the body up and twisting off the feet. Ask the children to see how far they can turn around using this particular method. Turns should be attempted to both the left and the right and each one should end in a controlled two-footed landing.

2. Turn with the arms

A more controlled and stylish method of turning the body in a jump is by using the swing of one or both arms to create momentum to take the body around. Each child should stand upright with his arms above his head. He then tries to turn to the left by jumping and simultaneously swinging his right arm down, across his body and up again to join the left. Using this method, the children should be able to make controlled quarter, half and even full turns.

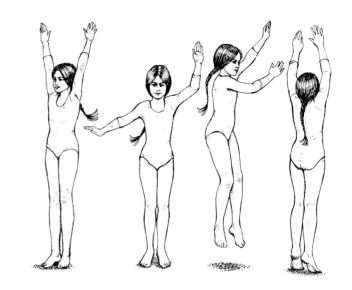

Flight turn with the arms.

3. Arms out, arms in

To demonstrate how the arms can affect turns of the body, ask the children to jump and turn, first with their arms outstretched and then with them tucked in to their chests. Ask the children if they notice any difference in the speed of turning or in how far they turn. With older pupils a discussion can follow on how the arms can be used to influence turns and how body shape in general might affect turns in the air.

4. One foot to the other

In this activity the children take off from one foot and make a half turn in the air to land on the other foot. Turns should be tried to the left and the right off both feet. Ask the children if it is easier or if they turn further when turning in a particular direction off each foot.

When the children show proficiency in landing on one foot the activity can be tried with a running take-off.

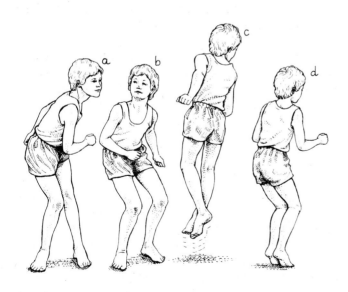

Jumping with a twist.

50

Main theme: apparatus work

SUITABLE APPARATUS: Springboards, benches, balancing planks, stools, boxes, platforms and mats to be used where indicated.

The height of the apparatus used will be dependent upon the age and the proficiency of the children but it should be predominantly low with one or two higher pieces available in activities where the movement is off the apparatus.

1. Mat jumping

In this activity the children can work two or three to a mat.

(i) Ask the children to find different ways of jumping over their mat, or over the corners. They must try to avoid touching it with their feet.

(ii) After the children have explored ways of jumping over their mat, let them repeat the activity but tell them that they must try to recross the mat each time from the position in which they land. Movement on the floor is not allowed.

(iii) Finally, ask the pupils to find different ways of crossing their mat such that they are always facing it on landing. Different combinations of one-footed and two-footed take-offs and landings should be encouraged in this activity.

2. Turn off the apparatus

Using a standing, two-footed take-off from a piece of apparatus the children jump and try making a quarter turn in the air to land on a mat. The importance of completing the turning movement in flight must be stressed in order that a controlled two-footed landing can be made on the mat. The children should slowly build up to making half turns in the air, in order to come down facing their apparatus, and then to full three hundred and sixty turns. USE BENCHES, BOXES, STOOLS, PLATFORMS AND MATS.

3. Turn on, turn off

Ask the children to stand next to a piece of apparatus and to try getting onto it first with a stepping movement and then with a jumping movement and each time to include a turn in the air. Movement off the apparatus should be in a similar way, with a controlled landing onto a mat. The stepping exercise could follow the pattern of the floorwork activity 'One foot to the other', with the children making a half turn onto the apparatus and a half turn off in order to complete a full three hundred and sixty degree turn in the movement. USE BENCHES, VERY LOW PLATFORMS, AND MATS.

4. Turn over the apparatus

This activity should be reserved for those children who show control and confidence in jumping onto apparatus.

The pupils stand facing a piece of apparatus and jump over it with a turn in the air in an attempt to be still facing it on landing. Jumps should be off two feet and if the pupils maintain good control they should be able to keep their feet together throughout the movement.

This activity could be combined with the previous one, with the pupils being asked to develop a short sequence which includes movements onto and off and also over the apparatus. USE BENCHES, VERY LOW PLATFORMS, AND MATS.

5. Run to turn

The greatest difficulty in performing movements in flight from a running take-off lies in the control of forward speed on landing. The children should therefore use minimal running speed when taking off in this activity as it is height, rather than distance travelled in flight, which is important to completing movements in the air.

Ask the children to run and take off from a piece of apparatus and to try completing half turns in the

air in order to face the apparatus on landing. The children should use only a three or a four stride approach to the apparatus and they should try both one-footed and two-footed take-offs.

Because of the problem associated with landing in this activity, control of this part of the movement should be stressed. It would also be appropriate to revise the safety roll technique of escaping from bad landings as a part of the activity. USE SPRINGBOARDS, VERY LOW BALANCING PLANKS AND MATS.

6. Turn and roll sequence

Ask the children to develop a sequence which includes three jumps from a piece of apparatus, each of which shows a different turning movement in flight and with the linking movements back to the apparatus being in the form of different rolls. USE BENCHES, STOOLS, BOXES, PLATFORMS AND MATS.

Concluding activities

1. Tag over a mat

For this activity the children work in pairs around a mat with one partner trying to 'tag' the other. The pupils start on opposite sides of their mat with neither of them being allowed to touch the mat and with both of them having to move by jumping or stepping over the mat or across its corners, walking and running not being allowed. Another rule which can be introduced is to forbid all turning movements other than those performed when crossing the mat. In this, if a pupil lands facing away from the mat then he must jump sideways or backwards, turns on the floor not being allowed.

This is a very demanding activity and only fifteen seconds should be allowed before the pupils are given a rest, after which the pupils can change roles.

2. Stepping stones

Arrange the mats about the floor and sufficiently close that the pupils may step from one to another. The children must then try to move to every mat and, if possible, cross each mat only once. The children should keep a count of how many mats they cross in travelling to every one in order to see who crosses the fewest and which is the most direct path to take.

With older pupils the activity can be made a little more demanding by allowing only a single contact by each foot when crossing a mat. This will eliminate 'long jumping' between the mats, improve movement control and extend the pupils' thinking in deciding upon the shortest route around the maze.

3. Turn left, turn right, turn about

In this activity the children stand in spaces and have to obey the teacher's commands, which are; 'Turn to the left', 'Turn to the right', and 'Turn about' meaning a one hundred and eighty degree turn. The children have to move each time by jumping and turning in the air, keeping their two feet together.

The activity can be used as an elimination game at the end of a lesson whereby the pupils who move incorrectly or who lose control, together with the pupil who moves last, are eliminated.

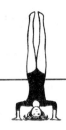

Points and areas of balance

Work in this theme is concerned with the basic principles of balance and with exploring the many possibilities for finding different balance positions. The main emphasis within the activities is on developing control skills, both in holding balance positions and in transferring from one balance position to another. Work concerned with body shape in balance comes in a later theme.

Weight can be supported on a variety of body parts and to avoid formalizing the work by introducing specific skill words such as handstand or headstand, it is better to talk in terms of 'areas of balance' when the weight is on large body areas such as the shoulders, back, bottom or front and 'points of balance' when the body is supported by the hands, knees, elbows, feet or other smaller body areas. This terminology will help the children to experiment more freely with the balance concept.

A good starting point with older children is to consider the meaning of the word 'balance'. In this the children should understand that the body is supported from below, as distinct from hanging positions where points of support are above the body, and that implicit in the word balance is the notion of stillness.

Introductory activities

1. Three, two, one

The children walk or jog around the floor and when the teacher calls a number, for instance 'Three', they must stop and adopt a position where they are balanced on that number of points.

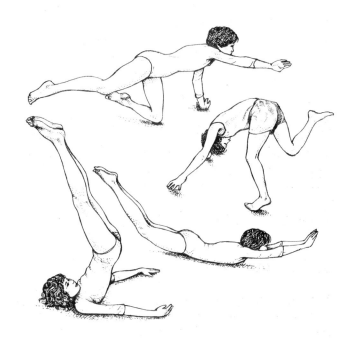

2. Points and areas across a mat

In this activity the children have to cross a mat by taking their weight on points of the body and return by moving on a large body area. Each time the children cross the mat they should try to use different points or a different body area. They could be asked to cross the mat and return four times in this way . This activity is particularly useful in establishing the terms 'body points' and 'body areas' in readiness for the floorwork and apparatus activities.

Main theme: floorwork

1. Find three balances

This activity can take two forms, the first to highlight the nature of balancing, and the second to focus attention more closely on which parts of the body can be considered as 'points' and which as 'areas'.

(i) As an introductory activity to the principles of balance the children can be asked to simply find three different balance positions. Emphasis should be on stillness, and unsteady positions, however difficult they might appear, should be rejected. The essence of balancing is control, and the children should be asked to hold each balance position for three or four seconds until the teacher says, 'Relax'.

(ii) This activity can be repeated with the children being asked to find balances alternately on body areas and body points. Their attention should be drawn to the many different parts of the body that can be used for supporting their weight. This is best done by asking different children to demonstrate the balances that they have found. USE MATS.

2. Transfer of weight

As important as steadiness in balancing is control in moving into or out of a balance, this activity emphasizes this particular aspect of movement.

Ask the children to select two balance positions and to move directly from one to the other. After they have practised this transfer they can be asked to do it slowly and then, as a focus on control, to move only when they receive a signal from the teacher. In this, the children should move into the first balance position and hold it until given the signal to change, whereupon they should move slowly into their second balance. This movement should be slow and precise, and the second balance should also be held until the teacher gives the signal to relax.

3. Balance on a given number of points

This activity contributes significantly to body awareness in that the children have to identify body points and select a given number in order to perform their balances.

Ask the children to find three different balances where the body is supported on three points. The same three body points may be used for each balance or different groups of points could be used. With older children it is worthwhile spending time considering stability factors and how best to arrange the points of balance for positions involving two, three and four points; for example, arranging three points in the form of a triangle rather than in a straight line. Such discussion is valuable in helping the children to work out for themselves how they might overcome problems in holding balance positions.

After practising their three balances, the children could try putting them together in a sequence. In this the means used in the previous activity for emphasizing control, where the teacher directs the movement, could again be employed.

Developments of this activity could include asking the children to extend their sequences by introducing further balances, or the number of body points to be used in the balances could be changed. USE MATS.

4. Points and areas sequence

To consolidate the ideas covered in the previous activities, a sequence of four balances, two using body points and two on body areas, is a good activity to include at the end of a period of floorwork in this theme. The principles of control in balancing and in transferring between balances can be reinforced and the extent of this control can be checked by the teacher directing movement through the sequence. This can be done by calling 'Change', to signal when the children should transfer from one balance to the next.

Shape in flight

The skil
many ar
work in
that chil
moveme
develop

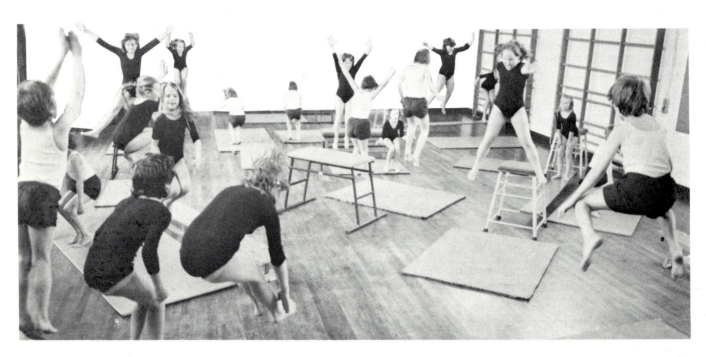

It is important for children to think of flight as a separate phase of movement from the take-off and the landing. Shapes or movements performed in the air should be initiated and completed during the flight phase and they should have little influence upon the other two elements.

The performance of any movement during flight requires time and this time is dependent upon the height achieved in jumping. This should be stressed as a means of encouraging pupils to work for maximum lift in their take-off. The early introduction of apparatus will also benefit the development of ideas and movement skills in this theme as jumps from apparatus give the pupils sufficient time to complete shapes prior to landing, something which they might find difficult when jumping off the floor.

It is essential, for safety reasons, that pupils adopt a correct position when landing. In concentrating on the performance of a shape, pupils can sometimes land whilst coming out of a movement. Sufficient practice should therefore be given in adopting simple shapes in the air in order that each pupil appreciates the time that they are in flight, in this way they will be better able to assess what shapes to attempt in the time available to them.

Main theme: apparatus work

SUITABLE APPARATUS: Benches, platforms, stools and boxes. Mats draped over the benches will provide a more comfortable work surface and will encourage a wider variety of balances on the benches.

In order that the children can build up confidence in performing balances and in transferring between balances on the apparatus, it is best to begin with an arrangement of variously sized flat surfaces. Only when the children fully appreciate the principles of balance and are performing with control should climbing frames and beams be introduced. Otherwise such apparatus will inevitably encourage the children to use positions which do not conform to the ideas being promoted within this theme, such as hanging positions.

1. Balance on body points

The children should first be allowed to explore this idea on a single piece of apparatus of their own choosing. In this way they can build up confidence by working at a level where they feel safe.

If this activity is used immediately after a floorwork activity involving points of balance the children could be asked to repeat their floor balances on the piece of apparatus. However, the children might require some guidance in selecting their piece of apparatus if this is done, to ensure that it is appropriate for the balances that they are to perform.

2. Balance on body areas

This activity follows the same format as the previous one and can again be used to follow a similar floorwork activity. Ask the children to find three different balances, emphasizing that the positions selected must be held quite still.

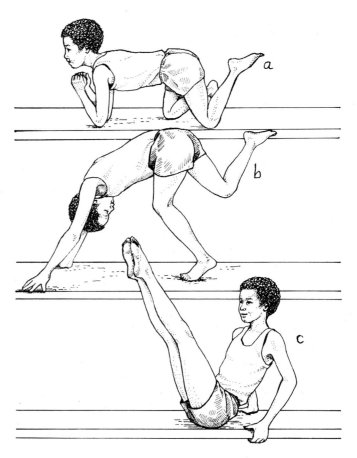

A three balance sequence on apparatus.

3. Sequence on the apparatus

Ask the children to find three balances on a piece of apparatus, two using body points and one on a body area, and to try to link them together in a sequence.

The difficulty in this activity lies in the selection of appropriate linking movements as the children will not be able to travel very far in transferring from one balance to the next. They should be encouraged to move slowly and smoothly through their sequence.

55

4. Sequence around the apparatus

In this activity the children use a piece of apparatus and the floor space around it for performing a sequence of balances. Ask the children to find just three balances with the first and third being on the floor and the second one on the apparatus. This will involve the children in moving both onto and off the apparatus during the sequence.

Aspects of work from other themes will need to be included in this activity to provide linking movements, and for these the children can be encouraged to use rolls and jumps to transfer between the different balance positions. The focus within this activity should again be on steadiness in balancing and also on control and smoothness of movement in transferring between balances.

This activity can be developed by introducing more specific instructions regarding the types of balance to be used, whether on body points or body areas, as well as the forms of linking movements to be used. The sequence could also be extended by including more balances or by introducing further pieces of apparatus.

5. Balance on all the apparatus

In this activity the children move to each piece of apparatus in turn to perform a balance. The teacher should direct the activity, waiting until everyone is holding a balance position before giving the signal to move on to the next piece of apparatus. The route around the apparatus can be determined by the teacher, or left for the children to choose for themselves. The latter does benefit the children's spatial awareness, particularly if a limit is imposed on the number of pupils allowed on each piece of apparatus.

Developments within this activity can focus upon several areas. The children can be asked to perform balances on a particular number of points or, to alternate balances between body points and body areas, linking movements could be limited to rolls or movements on the hands. Even the method of getting onto and off the apparatus can be highlighted by asking for jumps, jumps with turns or even rolling movements.

Concluding activities

1. Rolling statues

The children move about the floor off their feet by rolling, crawling or sliding until the teacher calls 'Freeze'. On this signal the children must try to hold the position they are in until they are told to carry on. This activity can be used as an elimination game at the end of a lesson with pupils who move when they are supposed to be still being given out.

2. The same is out

The teacher stands with his back to the class and gives the signal, 'Balance on points' or 'Balance on areas'. After giving a moment for the pupils to assume balance positions he then turns round, calling at the same time particular parts of the body, for example 'Hands and knees' or 'Elbows and feet'. If the activity is used as an elimination game then those pupils who are in balance positions on these parts of the body would be given out, or lose a life. The teacher can decide for himself how exact the match must be between the call and the body parts used for a life to be lost.

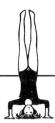

Shape in balance

The emphasis in this theme is on body shape when holding positions of balance and, just as in the theme 'Curling and stretching', attention should be drawn to all the limbs in the work in an attempt to increase the children's general body awareness.

The concept of symmetry in body shape, which again appears in the work on curling and stretching, can also be used in this theme and the children can be introduced to the idea of the different levels at which work can be performed, these being:

1. Low level: close to the floor.
2. Medium level: crouched or bent positions.
3. High level: upwardly extended positions.

Work in this theme draws on many ideas and concepts covered in the previous themes. In order to give the children a definite focus in their selection

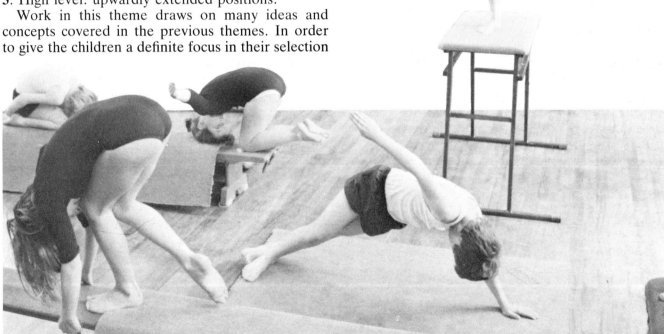

and organization of movement forms, the various concepts relating to shape, work level and balance must be introduced in a very precise way. It would be very easy for children to become confused when working on activities in this theme as there are so many variables which can influence their movement. The activities included are therefore designed to structure the children's thinking, yet still encourage a full exploration of movement ideas within the theme.

Introductory activities

The ideas and principles concerned with body shape in the themes of 'Curling and stretching' and 'Shape in flight', together with aspects of balance covered in the previous chapter, are very important to work here. Revision of principles and the use of floorwork activities from these themes would therefore form a most appropriate introduction to lessons in this theme.

1. Moving bridges

In this activity the children move about the floor off their feet by rolling, crawling or sliding and when the teacher calls 'Bridge', they must form a bridge-shaped balance. This call can be altered to 'High bridge', 'Long bridge' or 'Low bridge' to vary the shapes used by the children.

2. Over the bridge, under the bridge

Working in pairs each pupil in turn makes a low bridge shape which his partner must step or jump over and then pass under without touching. The activity can be made more demanding by asking each pupil to perform the movement three times in succession, and more vigorous by asking to see the first pair to finish. USE MATS.

Main theme: floorwork

1. Stretch and grow

This activity introduces the idea of working at different levels.

Ask the children to find three stretched balances using body points where the first is performed low down close to the floor, the second at a medium height level, and the third with the body making a high shape. Because of the three variables involved, (level, shape, and balancing on body points) the children will need to be reminded of the various task requirements as they work.

After practising their balances the children can try to put them together to form a sequence. Movement through the sequence could be directed by the teacher as a means of focusing attention upon control, the children only transferring from one balance to the next when the teacher gives the signal to change. USE MATS.

2. Stretch, tuck, stretch

Again using body points for balancing, the children find two stretched shapes and one tucked shape and perform them in the order stretch, tuck, stretch. To emphasize control in balancing and in transferring between balances and teacher can again direct the movement by indicating when to change.

The idea of working at different levels can be included in this activity, with the children first being asked to find stretched shapes which are close to the floor and then to repeat the activity using stretched shapes which extend upwards from the floor. USE MATS.

3. Stretched, curled and twisted

To introduce variety into the children's thinking about body shape in balance, ask them to look for other, interesting shapes where they use the ideas of curling and twisting to form balance positions. The balances should again be on body points with the children selecting their best or favourite three to combine into a sequence.

Both this activity and activities 1 and 2 could be repeated, or alternatively used, with the children performing their balances on body areas rather than points. USE MATS.

4. Six balance sequence

Older pupils can work towards the development of more complex sequences which include many balance positions and a wide variety of movement ideas. In developing a six balance sequence the children should try to work at all three levels, with perhaps two balances at each, to use both body points and body areas in balancing and to perhaps include both symmetrical and asymmetrical shapes. Thought must also be given to the selection of appropriate linking movements which allow for a smooth and controlled transfer between the balances. USE MATS.

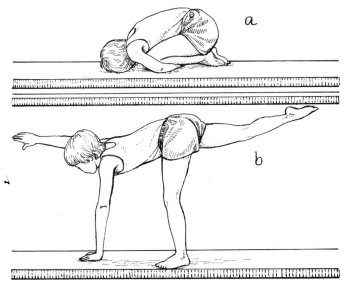

Stretch and curl on apparatus.

Main theme: apparatus work

SUITABLE APPARATUS: Benches, stools, boxes, beams, balancing planks, platforms and other apparatus which provides a flat working surface.

Each of the activities in the floorwork section could also be used and developed on the apparatus. Transferring floorwork sequences onto the apparatus serves to consolidate balance and shape ideas tried in the floorwork, as well as focusing the children's attention on the need for control.

1. Stretch and curl on the apparatus

Working on a piece of apparatus of their own choosing, the children find two balances, one with a stretched shape and one in a curled position. They then practise moving from one to the other, moving as slowly as possible and holding the balances for at least three seconds. The teacher can finally direct this activity with calls of 'Stretch', 'Transfer' and 'Tuck', to lay emphasis on control and smoothness in the movement.

When the children show confidence and control in their movement, the activity can be developed with the addition of extra balances or with the children being required to use particular types of balances, for example on body points only, or at a low level on the apparatus.

2. Balance around the apparatus

In this activity the children work around a single piece of apparatus, using both the floor and the apparatus as support surfaces for balancing on. Ask the children to find three balances, two on the floor and one on the apparatus, and to combine the three into a sequence where they move from the floor onto the apparatus and off again. Having found suitable balances, the children must give thought to the selection of linking movements which allow them to transfer onto and off the apparatus smoothly and also enable them to move directly into their balance positions.

This activity can be developed by asking the children to include further balances, to use particular shapes in their balances or to use certain linking movements.

3. Directed balances around the apparatus

This activity lays particular emphasis upon control with the teacher directing both the children's movement between the pieces of apparatus and the shapes that they are to use when balancing on the apparatus. These directions can be quite simple and for younger pupils need be no more than to ask the children to move slowly onto a piece of apparatus to perform a stretched balance and from there to move to another piece of apparatus to perform a tucked balance. However, with older pupils and the more able gymnasts the amount and the complexity of direction can be increased to include ways of moving between the apparatus as well as the types of balance to be used. For example, 'Roll to the next piece of apparatus and perform a stretched balance on three body points' or, 'Move to the apparatus without using your feet and perform a tucked balance on one body area'. Each of these sets of directions should be given whilst the children are holding their balance positions.

Concluding activities

This theme provides an ideal opportunity for introducing partner work to the children. In this the principle motive is for two children to work closely together in formulating a movement sequence. The intention at this stage is not for one partner to support the other in the performance of balances and, for safety reasons, this form of activity should not be allowed.

If these partner activities prove successful, the children could try to develop the ideas in the apparatus work of later lessons in this theme.

1. Partner balances

This activity could take two forms:
(i) The children, working in pairs, try to develop a sequence of three balances which they can perform simultaneously with both the balance shapes and the linking movements being as near identical as possible.
(ii) An alternative, which may appeal to the older and the more able gymnasts, is the development of a sequence where the movements of the two partners are complementary to each other. For example, whilst one partner performs a low balance the other may adopt a high balance position and as one moves down to the next position the other moves up. The movements and balances of the two partners are still performed simultaneously but the match is in the nature of the differences rather than the similarities. USE MATS.

2. Mirror image

This activity can also take two forms:
(i) At a simple level the activity involves one pupil in moving very slowly from one balance position into another, with a partner trying to follow these movements as closely as possible.
(ii) A more difficult variation, and one which the older pupils might enjoy, is where one pupil performs a simple routine of moving from one balance into another whilst a partner tries to perform the routine in front or alongside as if he were the mirror image of the performer. The children will have fun deciding how the image would appear. Indeed, this activity could lead into or fit nicely into work being done in the classroom on mirrors and reflected images. USE MATS.

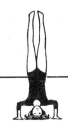

Balance work upon the hands

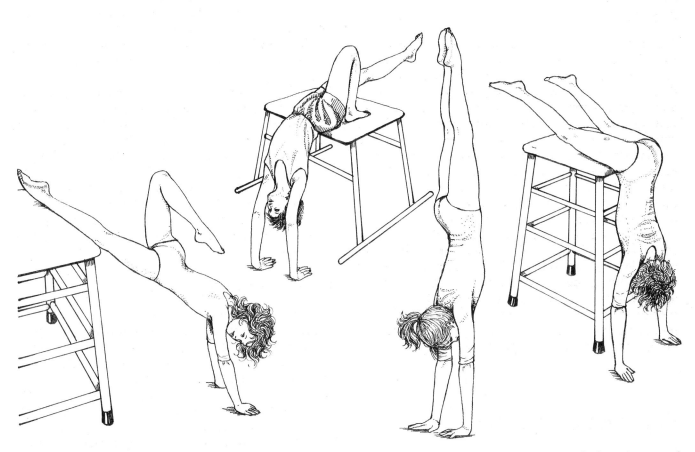

The ability to perform balances where support and control come principally from the hands is something of a landmark in gymnastics. Success in this skill area gives a child considerable confidence which will benefit his work in all the other areas.

This theme should be introduced after the other themes concerned with balance, and also after much work has been done on general movement utilizing the hands. The intention behind the work is to encourage pupils to take their weight increasingly upon their hands and to progress towards the eventual performance of a full hand balance.

Introductory activities

The introductory activities given in the theme 'Movement utilizing the hands' are equally acceptable as starting activities for lessons within this theme.

1. Chase around a clockface

Working in pairs, the children lie on their sides on a mat with their heads close together in the middle and their bodies facing opposite directions, like the hands of a clock reading twelve thirty. In this position the children raise themselves onto their hands and feet and on a signal from the teacher they both move clockwise, pivoting on their hands and each trying to catch the other before the teacher calls a halt. Only five seconds should be allowed for each chase and, after the pupils have had a brief rest, they can be set off again in an anti-clockwise direction. USE MATS.

2. Hand walk

In this activity the children support themselves on their hands in a press-up position but with the tops of their feet and not their toes on the floor. In this position the children walk with their hands and trail their bodies, seeing how many mats they can cross before they have to lie down for a rest. Alternatively, the children could be asked to try crossing all the mats and to count how many rests they have to take during the journey. USE MATS.

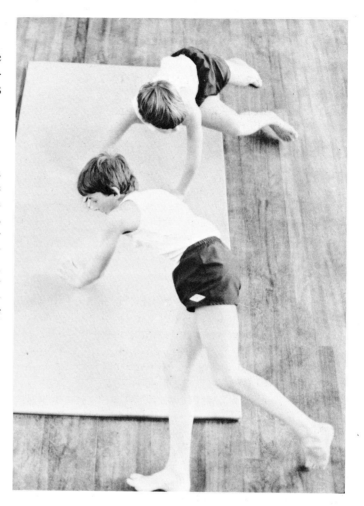

Above: Two partners in 'Chase around a clock-face'. Below: Movement by means of handwalking technique.

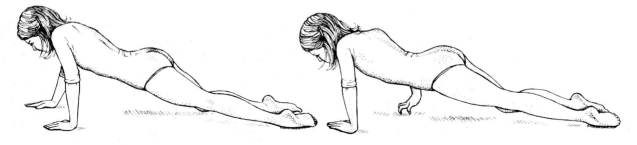

Main theme: floorwork

1. Balances including the hands

Ask the children to find three balance positions on body points where the hands are included as two of the points used. The pupils should be reminded of the balance factors of control and stillness as they work, and they should be encouraged to spread their fingers as this increases the effectiveness of the hands in controlling a balance. The three balances can then be combined into a sequence by the inclusion of linking movements. USE MATS.

2. Limited points

To increase the part played by the hands in holding balances, the previous activity can be repeated with a limit being placed on the number of body points to be used in the balance positions. For example, the children could be asked to use only three points of balance with two of these always being the hands. Again the balances can be combined to form a sequence by the introduction of linking movements. USE MATS.

3. Balances at different levels

In this activity all balances must again involve use of the hands, with the children having to find balance positions at the three different height levels for working. Emphasis in the activity should be on control and body shape in the balance positions adopted.
(i) Low level: Ask the children to find three balances where they form shapes very close to the floor.
(ii) Medium level: Ask the children to find three balances where their bodies are crouched or in half-standing positions.
(iii) High level: Ask the children to find three balances which show high or upwardly extended shapes.

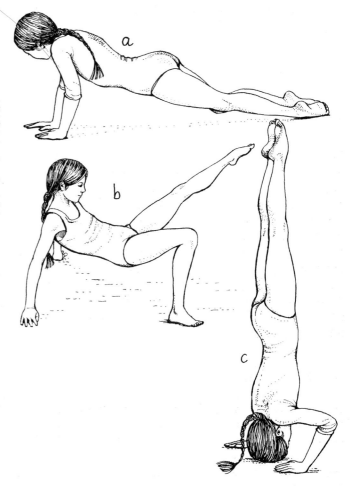

Balances at (a) low, (b) medium and (c) high levels.

The work at each level can be developed by asking the pupils to combine their balances into sequences, or a final three balance sequence could be developed with the children including one balance from each of the three levels. The work could also be made more difficult by limiting the number of body points that the children are allowed to use in balancing, although there will be a natural increase in the level of difficulty as the children are required to make increasingly higher balance shapes. USE MATS.

Main theme: apparatus work

SUITABLE APPARATUS: Boxes, benches, balancing planks, stools, platforms, beams and mats.

1. Floor balances on the apparatus

In most cases a balance using the hands which is performed on the floor can also be performed on apparatus, particularly if the apparatus provides a flat-topped working surface. A good introductory activity to apparatus work in this theme, where the children may be apprehensive about taking their weight upon their hands, is to ask the pupils to try performing three balances, which they have developed on the floor, on a piece of apparatus of their own choosing. This eliminates the need for the pupils to think too much about the actual nature of the balances, so allowing them to concentrate upon control factors.

A revision of the definition of a balance as a still position which is supported from below, may be necessary, as the children might otherwise include positions where there is an element of hanging, particularly when beams are being used.

2. Balance on and balance off

If the children's skill in balancing upon the hands is to develop, they must be encouraged to rely increasingly upon their hands for support when in balance positions. In this activity the children are asked to find three balances, each on three points, two where they are supported by their hands on the floor and one other part of the body which rests on or against the apparatus, and one balance using three body points, two of which must be the hands, actually on the apparatus.

When the children have explored this idea and practised their three balances, they can be asked to combine them to form a sequence where they move onto and off the apparatus. The first and third balances in the sequence will be those where the hands are on the floor, the second balance will be the one on the apparatus. The children will find it quite a challenging task to select linking movements which will enable them to move smoothly through their sequence, particularly if they are working on fairly high pieces of apparatus.

3. Sequence around the apparatus

The children should be given the opportunity to explore balance ideas within this theme on each of the pieces of apparatus. This can be provided by asking the children to develop a sequence where they use three different pieces of apparatus on which to perform balances. A preliminary exercise in the development of this sequence would be to allow the children to work on each piece of apparatus separately, in order to find three balances which they are happy with. They will then need to establish a route and find linking movements for transferring between the three pieces of apparatus.

To stress use of the hands in this work, the children can be asked to move across the floor by taking their weight on their hands and to use only two or three point balances on the apparatus, where two of the points must be the hands.

Having practised their sequences, the children should be asked to perform them with the teacher directing the movement. This would serve to emphasize control, both in the holding of the balance positions and in the transfer movements between the pieces of apparatus.

Concluding activities

In the final part of lessons in this theme, activities designed to increase arm strength, such as those given in the theme of 'Movement utilizing the hands', could be used. Alternatively, the time could be spent on practising handstanding.

1. The handstand

This skill needs to be built up in stages:
(**i**) The children should begin in a crouched position with their hands on the floor and drive one leg up into the air. This action provides the lift for both legs, and the pupils should continue practising until they can achieve steadiness on their hands.
(**ii**) The pupils next work towards full extension of the body with the trailing leg being brought up to join the other. Continued practice will allow the pupils to achieve a more upright position.

Partner support is very important in the development of handstanding skill. It provides the necessary stability to allow a pupil to feel what it is like to be in a handstand position, and it gives time for the development of balance control. Correct supporting involves being up close to the performer with the right leg against his right shoulder, or the left leg to the left shoulder and with the head tilted to the side in order to avoid the gymnast's feet. The supporter should steady the gymnast at the hips and *must not hold his legs*. The gymnast must be able to come down when he wishes, if he is held up by the supporter then he will ultimately collapse.

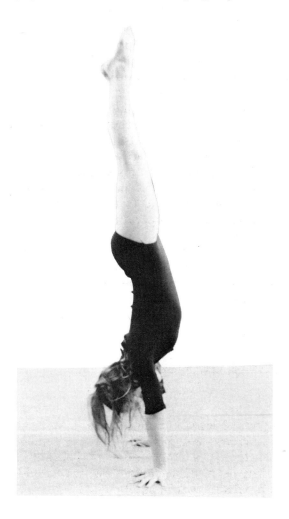

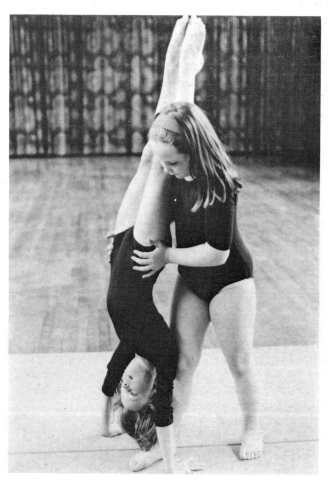

The children should be encouraged to come down from a handstand position one leg at a time, to walk out of the handstand. If both feet come down together, the landing is very heavy and a pupil could sustain injury. The supporter can help the gymnast to establish this habit by merely restraining one leg if he feels that both of them are dropping to the floor at the same time.

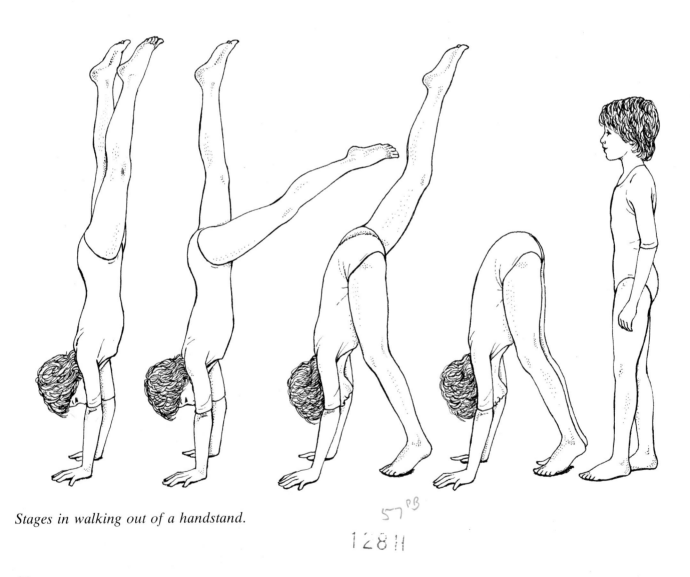

Stages in walking out of a handstand.